SOUS VIDE *Ketogenic* COOKBOOK

LOW-CARB, HIGH-FAT, SATISFYING SOUS VIDE RECIPES. THE ULTIMATE KETO COOKBOOK TO FIX YOUR METABOLISM, LOSE WEIGHT AND STAY HEALTHY.

Sophia Marchesi

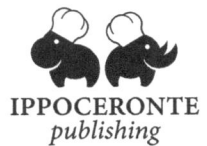

IPPOCERONTE
publishing

Copyright © 2021 by Sophia Marchesi
All rights reserved

This document is geared towards providing exact and reliable information with regards to the topic and issue covered. The publication is sold with the idea that the publisher is not required to render accounting, officially permitted, or otherwise, qualified services. If advice is necessary, legal or professional, a practiced individual in the profession should be ordered.

From a Declaration of Principles which was accepted and approved equally by a Committee of the American Bar Association and a Committee of Publishers and Associations.

In no way is it legal to reproduce, duplicate, or transmit any part of this document in either electronic means or in printed format. Recording of this publication is strictly prohibited and any storage of this document is not allowed unless with the written permission from the publisher. All rights reserved.

The information provided herein is stated to be truthful and consistent, in that liability, in terms of inattention or otherwise, by any usage or abuse of any policies, processes, or directions contained within is the solitary and utter responsibility of the recipient reader. Under no circumstances will any legal responsibility or blame be held against the publisher for any reparation, damages, or monetary loss due to the information herein, either directly or indirectly.

Respective authors own all copyrights not held by the publisher.

The information herein is offered for informational purposes solely and is universal as so. The presentation of the information is without a contract or any type of guarantee assurance.

The trademarks that are used are without any consent, and the publication of the trademark is without permission or backing by the trademark owner. All trademarks and brands within this book are for clarifying purposes only and are owned by the owners themselves, not affiliated with this document.

Cover designed by thiwwy design (@thiwwy).
Cover Photo by Ella Olsson (@ellaolsson) from Unsplash

CONTENTS

INTRODUCTION 7
RECIPES 11
1. Baked Yam Chips 12
2. Cauliflower 14
3. Flank Steak, Apricot, and Brie Bites 16
4. Cream of Celery Soup 18
5. Herbed Pork Chops 20
6. Tomatoes Stuffed with Tuna 22
7. Chicken Skewers 24
8. Lemongrass and Garlic Pork Belly Roll 26
9. Fresh Vegetables Confit 28
10. Okra and Spiced Yogurt 30
11. Parmesan and Scallion Omelet 32
12. Perfect Egg Tostada 34
13. Soft-Poached Eggs 35
14. Eggs with Roasted Peppers 36
15. Egg 38
16. Asparagus with Hollandaise 39
17. Flax Seeds Mix 40
18. Cider Dipped Fennel 42
19. Cinnamon and Egg Mix 43
20. Simple Mushroom Soup 44
21. Cauliflower Soup 46
22. Pork Chops with Mushrooms 48
23. Favorite Thai Dinner 50
24. Mid-Week Chicken 52
25. Pork Tenderloin 54
26. Lamb Chops with Basil Chimichurri 56

27. Chipotle Apple Pork Loin 58
28. French Duck Confit 60
29. Sausage Tomato 62
30. Spice Rubbed Short Ribs 64
31. Miso Soy Glazed Pork Chops 66
32. Indian Style Pork 68
33. Warm Beef Soup with Ginger 70
34. Perfectly Cooked Mushrooms 72
35. Tender Leeks with Herbed Butter 74
36. Parmesan Garlic Asparagus 76
37. Chili and Garlic Sauce 78
38. Turmeric Pickled Cauliflower 80
39. Garlic Dipping Sauce with Asparagus 82
40. Scallops with Lemon Herb Salsa Verde 84
41. Swordfish with Balsamic Brown Butter Sauce 86
42. Savory Halibut 88
43. Mezcal-Lime Shrimp 90
44. Poached Tuna with Basil Butter 92
45. Pecan Pie 94
46. Strawberry Mousse 96
47. Lemon Tart 98
48. Dark Chocolate Mousse 100
49. Crème Brûlée 102
50. Mini Strawberry Cheesecake Jars 104

TEMPERATURE CHARTS **106**
COOKING CONVERSION **112**
RECIPE INDEX **116**

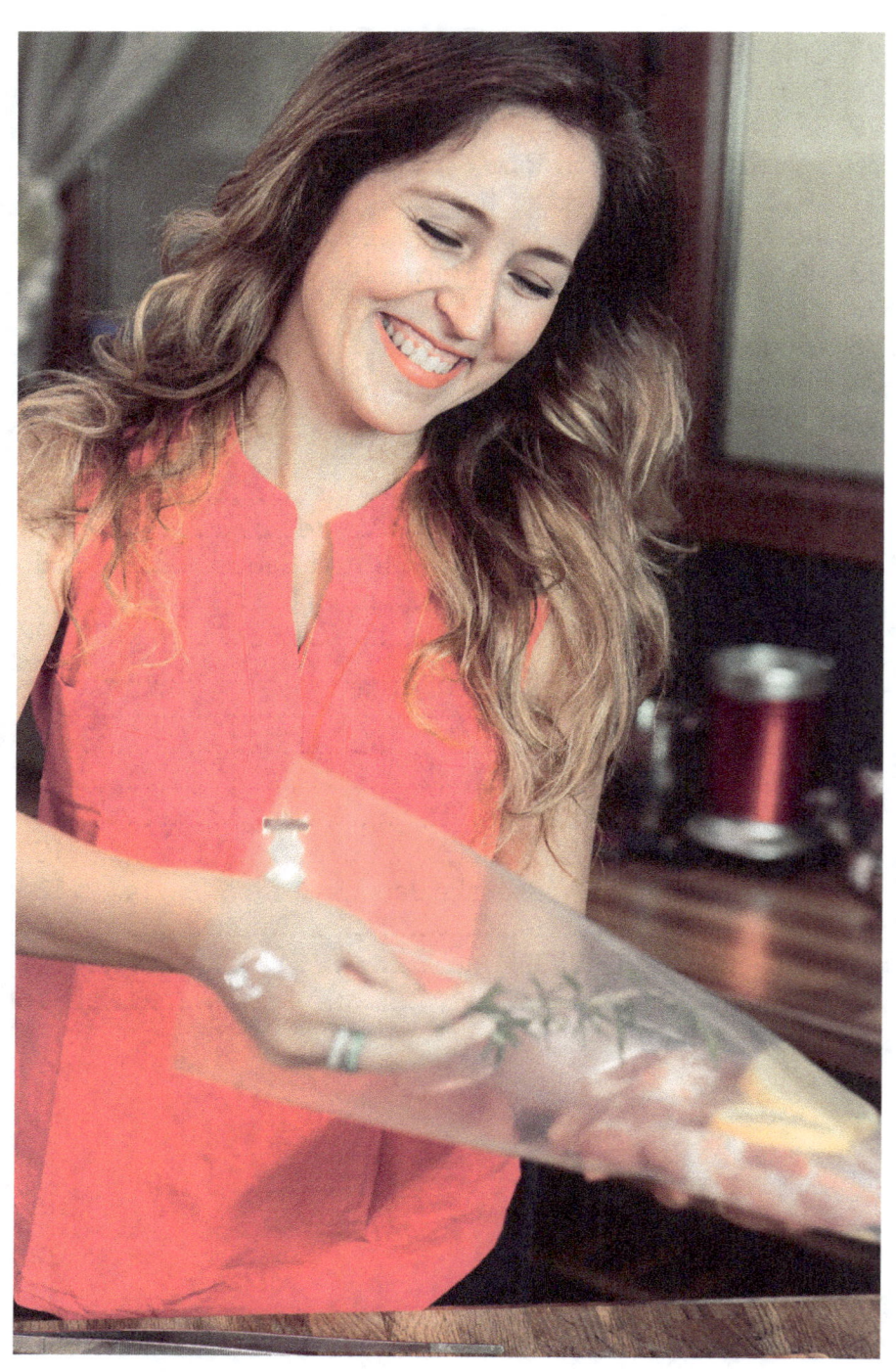

INTRODUCTION

Cooking is something that runs in my blood, most of my food memories are of my Nan cooking Sunday dinners - lasagna and cannelloni to share with the whole family. Since a young age, keeping my weight under control has always been a challenge. I am from an Italian-American family where eating healthy was not on the top of the priorities. It was not easy being the overweight girl at school but, learning more about food and its nutrients and becoming a professional chef helped me during my transformation. I have never liked to be stuck in a classroom, I started culinary school at a very young age, and the only thing I really wanted was to be out cooking. You could say I was not a particularly good student, but I have always been really passionate about good and healthy food.

I have been working in a professional kitchen since I was seventeen years old and I've been running my own restaurant since I was 23. The past thirty years have been a rewarding, yet arduous journey that I spent learning the basics and mastering the different cuisines and techniques by taking the best out of each of them.

Eating healthily it's not simple, we are surrounded by junk food and temptations. What I would like to share with you in this book is a diet and a cooking technique that changed my life! Keto diet and Sous Vide are a lethal combination that shreds all those extra pounds.

The ketogenic diet is a high-fat, adequate-protein, low-carbohydrate diet. The idea is for you to get more calories from protein and fat and less from carbohydrates. You cut back most on the carbs that are easy to digest, like sugar, soda, pastries, and white bread. Eating less than 50g of carbohydrates a day will lead to breaking down proteins and fats for energy. This process is called ketosis. The ketogenic diet is normally considered a short-term diet that will drastically help losing weight in a short period.

Sous Vide: This innovative cooking method is something my grandmother never thought existed and creates the perfect opportunity to spend some time in the kitchen with my family. For these reasons, I think the Sous Vide is the perfect combination of my professional and domestic life.

Sous Vide is the French term that translates to "under vacuum" and it is the method for preparing a dish at a specifically controlled temperature and time; your food should be prepared at the temperature at which it will be eaten. Put simply, this procedure involves placing food in vacuum seal bags and boiling it in a specially built bath of water for longer than average cooking times (usually 1 to 7 hours, up to 48 or more in some cases). Cooking at an exact temperature takes the guesswork out of the equation that defines a perfect meal. You can easily prepare your steak, chicken, lamb, pork, etc., exactly the way you like it, every single time.

It is easy to use and leads to great results every time. You will end up with food that is more tender and juicier than anything else you've ever made. This technique will help you to take your everyday cooking to a higher level. To make a top dish, most of the time, you do not need exotic ingredients, it is just a matter of getting the best from the ingredients you already know.

The greatest part of Sous Vide cooking is that it does not require your constant presence in the kitchen. When the food is sealed in a bag and placed in the water bath, you can leave it at a low temperature, and it will cook on its own without asking much of your attention. The Sous Vide Cookers that are nowadays available in the market are efficient at regulating the perfect temperature to cook food according to its texture while maintaining the minimum required temperature. So, while your food is in the water, your hands are practically free to work on other important tasks or spend some quality time with your family.

It is an artful skill that is definitely worth trying. If it is just your first time, don't feel bad if you don't get the results you wanted to achieve. You will get better by gaining experience with this cookbook! The key is having patience, the right information, and consistency.

The meals prepared with Sous Vide are tasty and healthy, since this technique does not use added fats during the preparation of your dish also, using low temperature ensures that the perfect cooking point is reached.

Dishes included in this cookbook are simple, delicious, and provide you with so many options that you'll be preparing them for years to come. These recipes are made to be shared with the people you love and to build new precious food memories as I did with my Nan.

RECIPES

1. BAKED YAM CHIPS

Cal.: 193 | Fat: 9g | Protein: 8g

Preparation Time: 12 minutes
Cooking Time: 90 minutes
Servings: 4

Ingredients

Coarse sea salt and freshly ground black pepper, to taste
1/3 teaspoon ancho chili powder
1 pound yams, peeled and cubed
½ teaspoon Hungarian paprika
2 tablespoons extra-virgin olive oil

Directions

1. Prepare your sous-vide water bath to a temperature of 183°F/84°C.

2. In a large bowl, sprinkle over yams with pepper and salt.

3. Transfer the yam to a Ziploc bag and seal it after squeezing out the excess air.

4. Immerse the bag into the water bath and cook for 1 hour.

5. Once cooked, remove the bag from the water bath and pat dry the yams using a kitchen towel.

6. Preheat your oven to 350°F/176°C.

7. Place the yams orderly on a parchment-lined baking sheet.

8. Sprinkle over with chili powder and Hungarian paprika and drizzle with olive oil.

9. Bake for 23 minutes and remove.

10. Serve and enjoy!

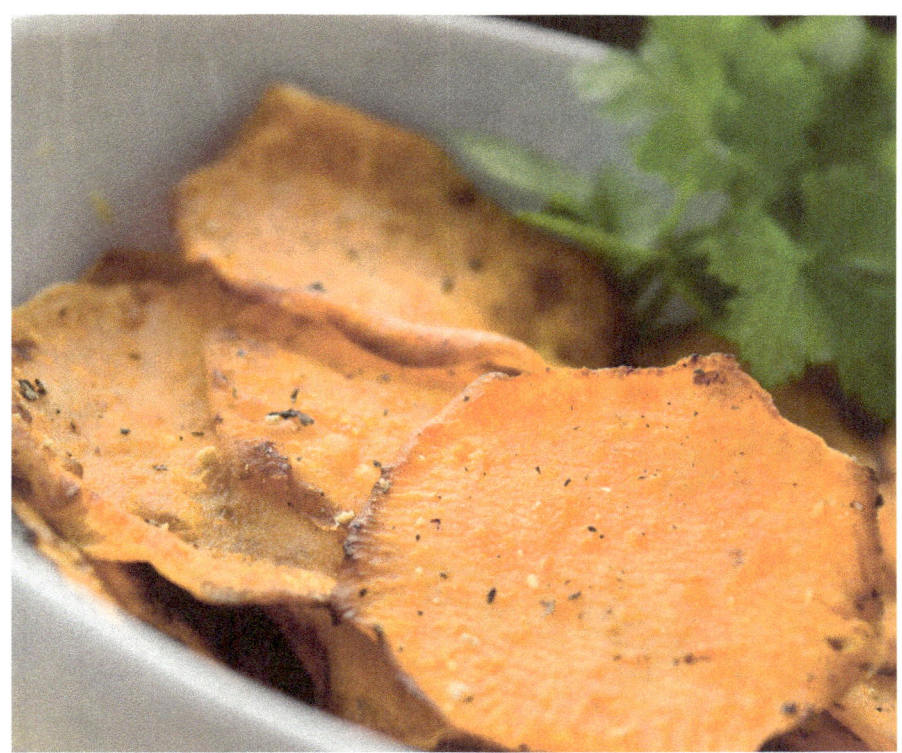

2. CAULIFLOWER

Cal.: 294 | Fat: 20g | Protein: 9g

Preparation Time: 8 minutes
Cooking Time: 50 minutes
Servings: 4

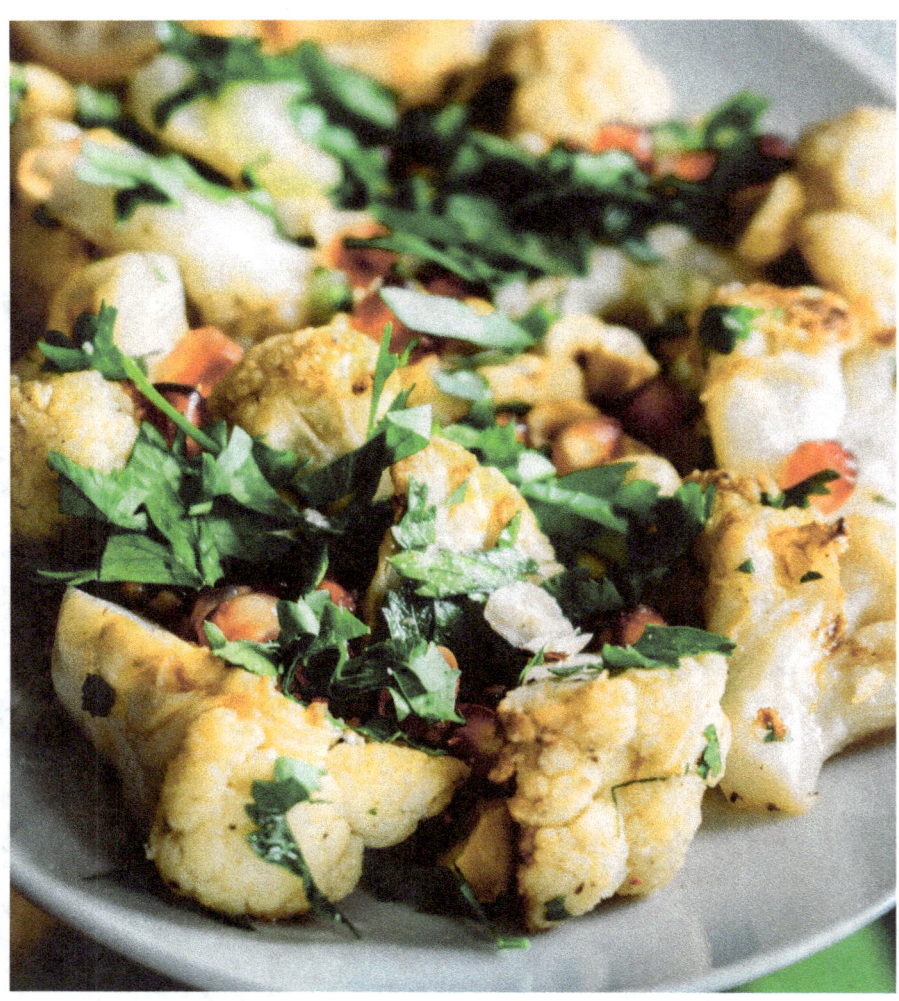

Ingredients

1 cauliflower
10 drops chili oil
Some chili butter
Some herb butter
2 tbsp. chives rings
1 pinch each white pepper, sea salt and nutmeg
Juice and zest of 1 untreated lemon

Directions

1. Put the cauliflower florets with salt, freshly ground nutmeg, chili oil and lemon juice and zest in a vacuum bag and vacuum seal.

2. Preheat the water bath to 144°F/62°C and cook the cauliflower for 50 minutes.

3. To finish, heat some chili and herb butter in the pan or wok. Take the cauliflower florets out of the bag and toss in the butter. Season if necessary and sprinkle with the chive's rings.

4. This buttery, aromatic cauliflower can be enjoyed as a side dish or as a stand-alone, vegetarian dish.

3. FLANK STEAK, APRICOT, AND BRIE BITES

Cal.: 549 | Fat: 31g | Protein: 16g

Preparation Time: 13 minutes
Cooking Time: 18 hours
Servings: 6

Ingredients

1 flank steak (about 2 pounds)
1 teaspoon sea salt
1 teaspoon freshly ground black pepper
1 teaspoon paprika
1 medium wheel Brie
10–12 dried apricots
20–24 fresh mint leaves

Directions

1. Fill the water bath with water. Set your machine temperature to 135°F/57°C.

2. Rub the flank steak all over with salt, pepper and paprika. Place the steak in a food-safe bag and vacuum seal the bag.

3. Place the steak in the water bath and cook for 12–18 hours.

4. Remove from the water bath and immediately place in an ice bath to chill the steak. Cut the flank steak, against the grain, into thin slices.

5. Cut the Brie cheese into small slices and cut the dried apricots in half.

6. Assemble the bites by placing a mint leaf and dried apricot half on a piece of sliced Brie. Wrap with a slice of flank steak and pierce with a toothpick. Keep them in the fridge until ready to serve.

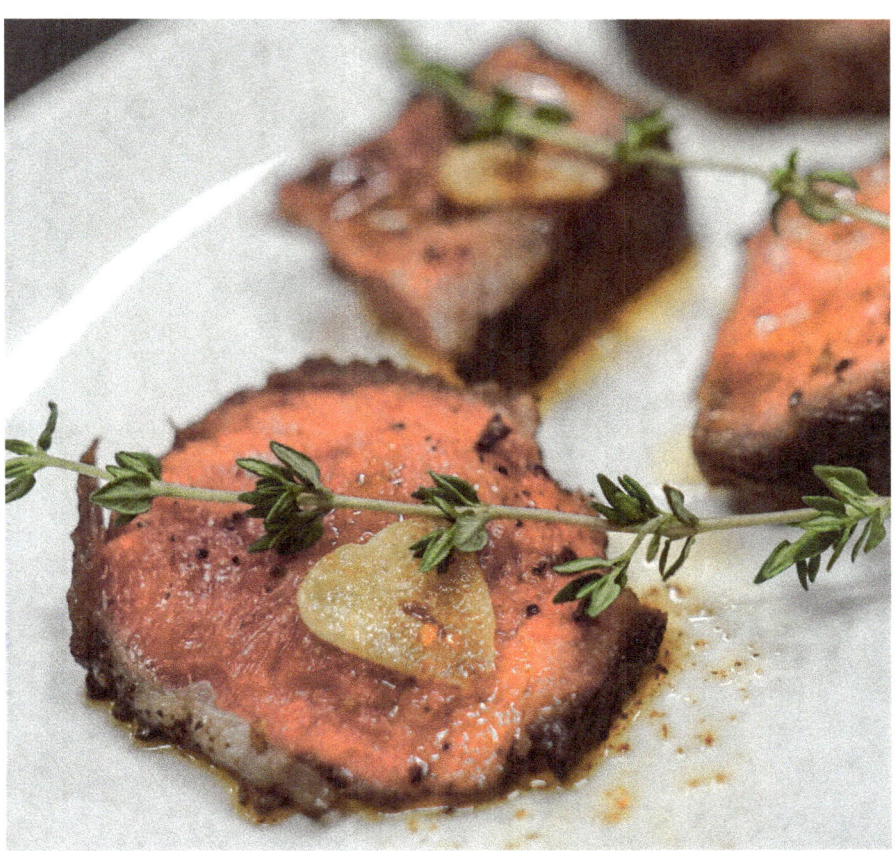

4. CREAM OF CELERY SOUP

Cal.: 372 | Fat: 23g | Protein: 14g

Preparation Time: 18 minutes
Cooking Time: 60 minutes
Servings: 2

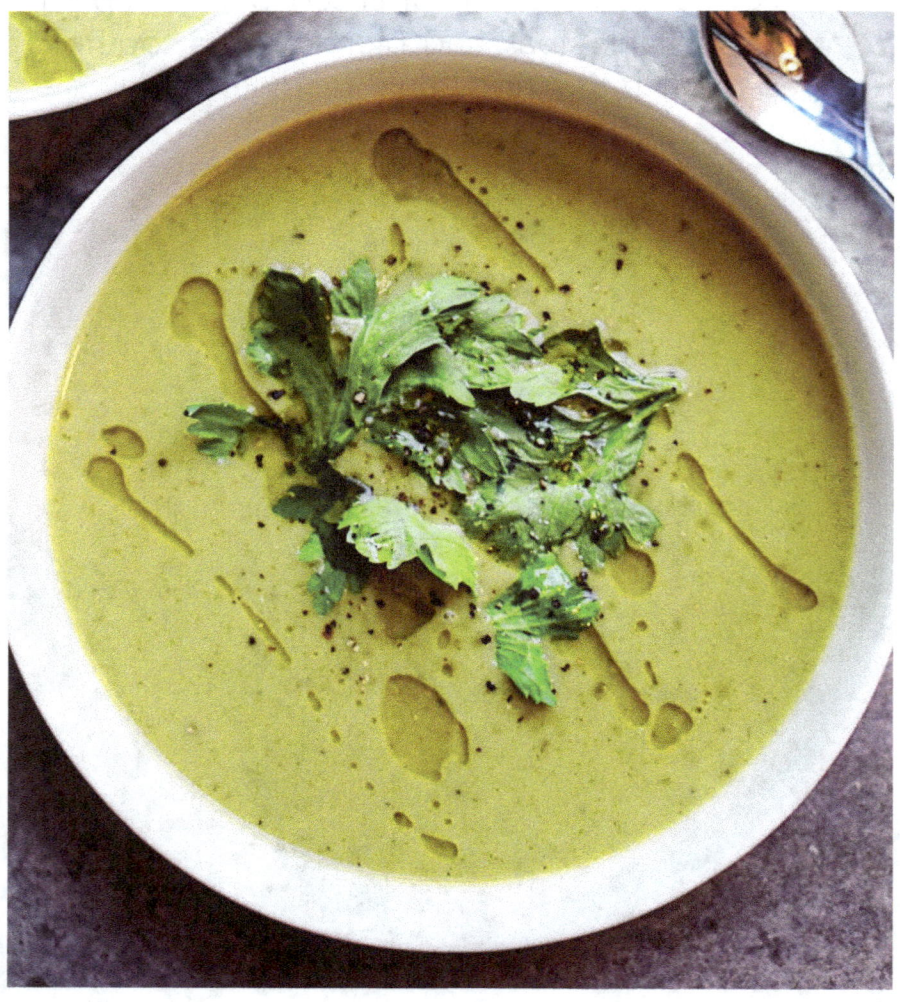

Ingredients

2 cups celery, diced into large pieces
½ cup russet potatoes, peeled, diced into small pieces
½ cup leek, diced into large pieces
½ cup stock (vegetable or chicken)
½ cup heavy cream
1 tablespoon butter
1 bay leaf
1 teaspoon kosher salt or to taste
White pepper powder to taste

Directions

1. Set your Sous Vide machine to 180°F/82°C.

2. Place all the ingredients in a Ziploc or a vacuum-seal bag. Remove the air by using the water displacement method or a vacuum-sealed one. Seal and then immerse in the water bath. Cook for 1 hour or until the vegetables are tender.

3. When done, remove the bay leaf and purée the soup. Strain through a wire mesh strainer and discard the solids. Serve hot.

5. HERBED PORK CHOPS

Cal.: 370 | Fat: 32.5g | Protein: 18.2g

Preparation Time: 11 minutes
Cooking Time: 1 hour
Servings: 4

Ingredients

4 bone-in pork chops
4 sprigs of fresh rosemary
2 garlic cloves, crushed
2 tablespoons olive oil
2 tablespoons butter
Salt and pepper

Directions

1. Heat your Sous Vide Machine to 140°F/60°C for medium-rare chops. For medium-well, set your Sous Vide Machine to 150°F/66°C.

2. Place the chops, herbs, salt, pepper, and butter in a vacuum-sealed bag.

3. Immerse in the water bath for at least 1 hour and not more than 4.

4. When the chops are nearly finished, heat a skillet

(preferably cast-iron) on high heat with olive oil.

5. Remove chops from the bag and sear quickly on both sides until a nice crust is achieved.

6. Remove from the pan and serve immediately.

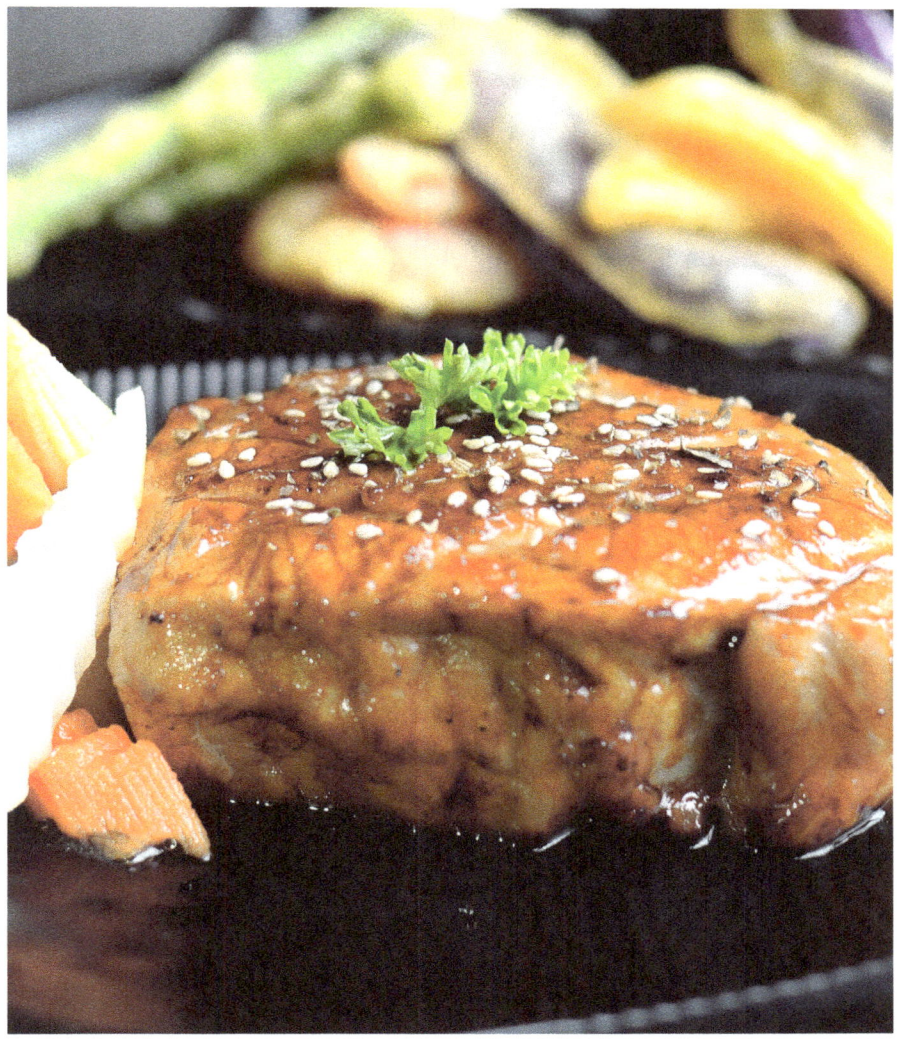

6. TOMATOES STUFFED WITH TUNA

Cal.: 162 | Fat: 32g | Protein: 18g

Preparation Time: 15 minutes
Cooking Time: 15 minutes
Servings: 5

Ingredients

4 tomatoes
2 cups white tuna
2 celery stalks
2 tablespoons capers
1 tablespoon olive oil
1 tablespoon red wine vinegar
½ cup parsley
Salt, pepper as per need

Directions

1. Preheat the Sous Vide machine to 195°F/91°C.

2. Take tuna is a Ziploc bag.

3. Place this bag in the water bath for 10 minutes.

4. Cut off the top and bottom thin slices of tomatoes. Remove the seeds and pulp using the spoon. Take

the seeds and pulp in a mixing bowl.

5. To this, add tuna, oil vinegar, celery, salt, pepper, capers, parsley and mix.

6. Cook this mixture for 5 minutes.

7. Add the tuna mixture into the tomato cavities and serve.

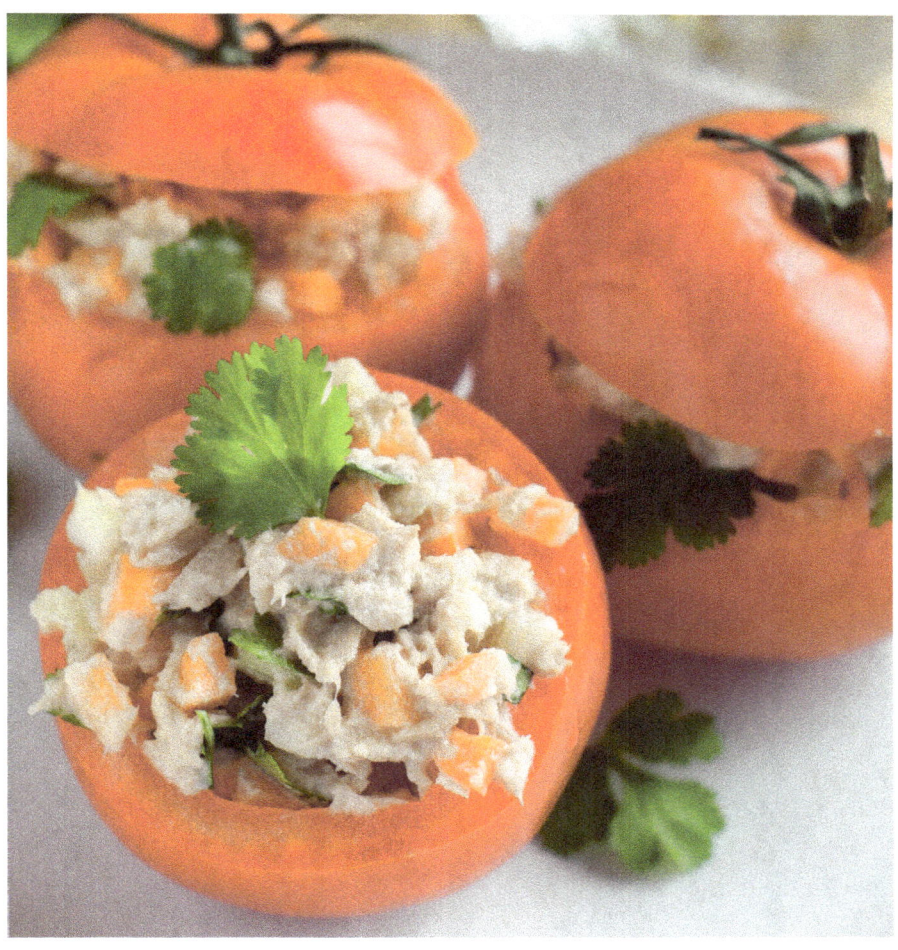

7. CHICKEN SKEWERS

Cal.: 298 | Fat: 12.1g | Protein: 35g

Preparation Time: 13 minutes
Cooking Time: 1 hours 45 minutes
Servings: 2

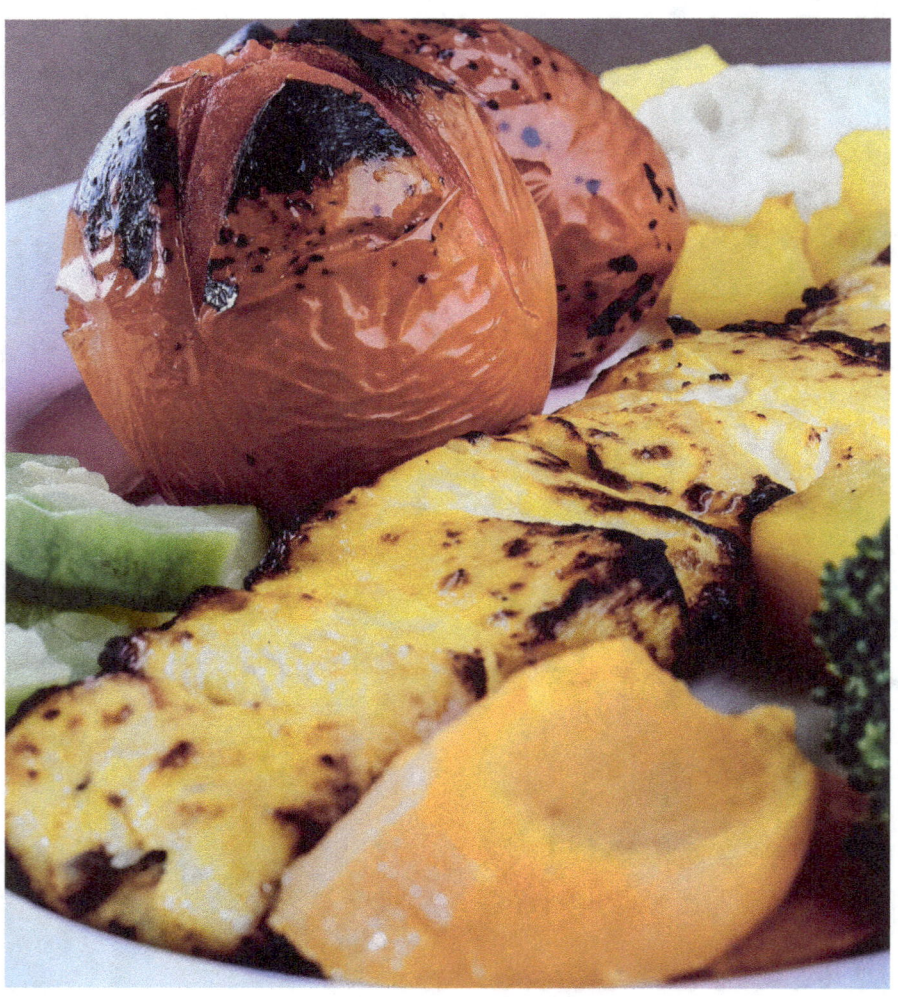

Ingredients

2 (4 oz.) chicken breasts, cubed
Salt, to taste
Black pepper, to taste
1 teaspoon cayenne pepper
½ teaspoon mustard powder
½ cup yogurt
1 tablespoon vegetable oil

Directions

1. Prepare and preheat the water bath at 150°F/65°C.

2. Mix chicken cubes with yogurt and all the spices in a bowl. Thread the chicken onto wooden skewers.

3. Place the skewers in two zipper-lock bags.

4. Seal the zipper-lock bags using the water immersion method. Immerse the sealed bag in the water.

5. Cover the water bath and cook for 1 hour, 15 minutes. Once done, remove the chicken skewers from the bag.

6. Grill the chicken skewers with oil in a grill pan for 1 minute per side.

7. Serve warm.

8. LEMONGRASS AND GARLIC PORK BELLY ROLL

Cal.: 439 | Fat: 28.9g | Protein: 35.5g

Preparation Time: 11 minutes
Cooking Time: 8 hours
Servings: 6

Ingredients

1 lb. pork belly, leave whole
3-½ teaspoons sea salt
½ teaspoon pepper
1/4 cup olive oil
4 stalks lemongrass, white part only
1 whole garlic bulb, peeled
2 bell peppers, sliced into strips
Cooking string to secure belly closed

Directions

1. Preheat the water bath to 165°F/74°C.

2. Generously season pork belly with salt all over.

3. Lay skin side down.

4. Add lemongrass, bell pepper, and garlic, in a line in the belly's center, and drizzle with a little olive oil.

5. Roll belly into a log and tie shut with a cooking string.

6. Add pork belly to a large bag.

7. Seal the bag and place in the preheated container.

8. Cook for 8 hours.

9. Slice into 1-inch-thick medallions and serve warm with your favorite sides.

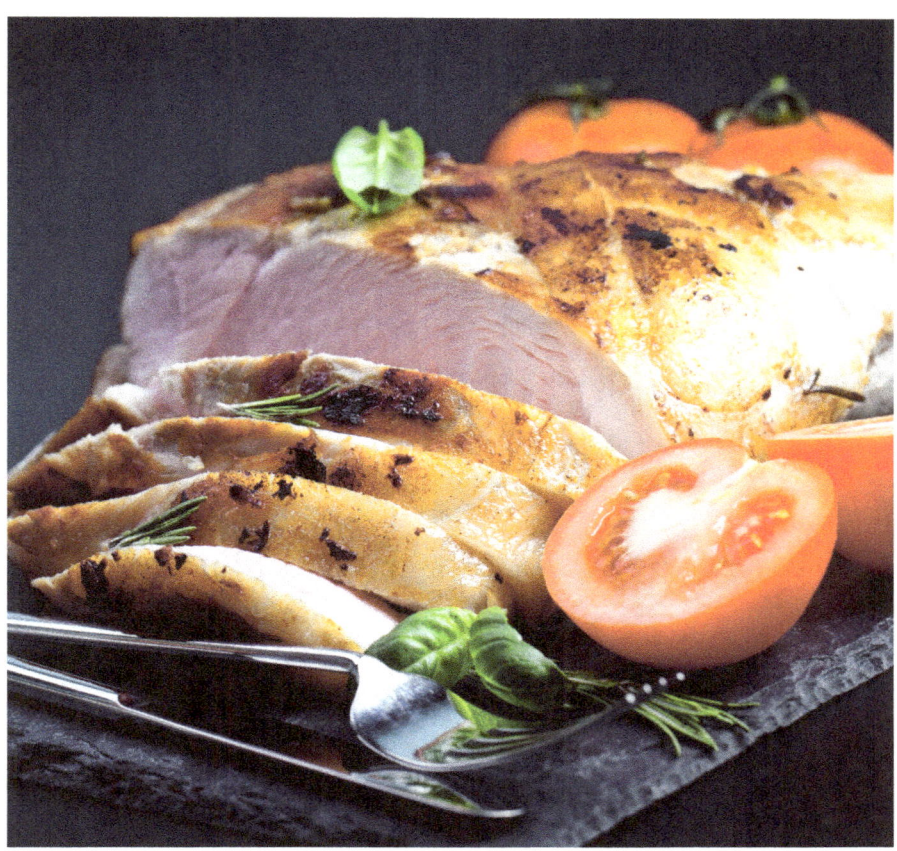

9. FRESH VEGETABLES CONFIT

Cal.: 387 | Fat: 31g | Protein: 19g

Preparation Time: 8 minutes
Cooking Time: 2 hours
Servings: 10

Ingredients

1 cup peeled pearl onions
1 cup peeled garlic cloves
6 cups olive oil
2 cups halved, deseeded mini peppers

Garnish:
10 to 12 ounces spreadable goat cheese
Keto bread slices, as required, toasted
Salt to taste
Fresh herbs of your choice

Directions

1. Preheat the Sous Vide machine to 185°F/85°C.

2. Place garlic in a Ziploc bag or vacuum-seal pouch. Pour 1½ cups oil into the pouch.

3. Add mini peppers into a second Ziploc bag. Pour 3 cups of oil into the pouch.

4. Add pearl onions into a third Ziploc bag. Pour 1½ cups oil into the pouch.

5. Vacuum seal the pouches.

6. Immerse the pouches in a water bath and adjust the timer for 1½ hours. When the timer goes off, remove the pouches from the water bath and place in chilled water for 30 minutes.

7. Spread goat cheese over toasted ciabatta slices. Top with vegetables from each pouch. Garnish with fresh herbs and serve.

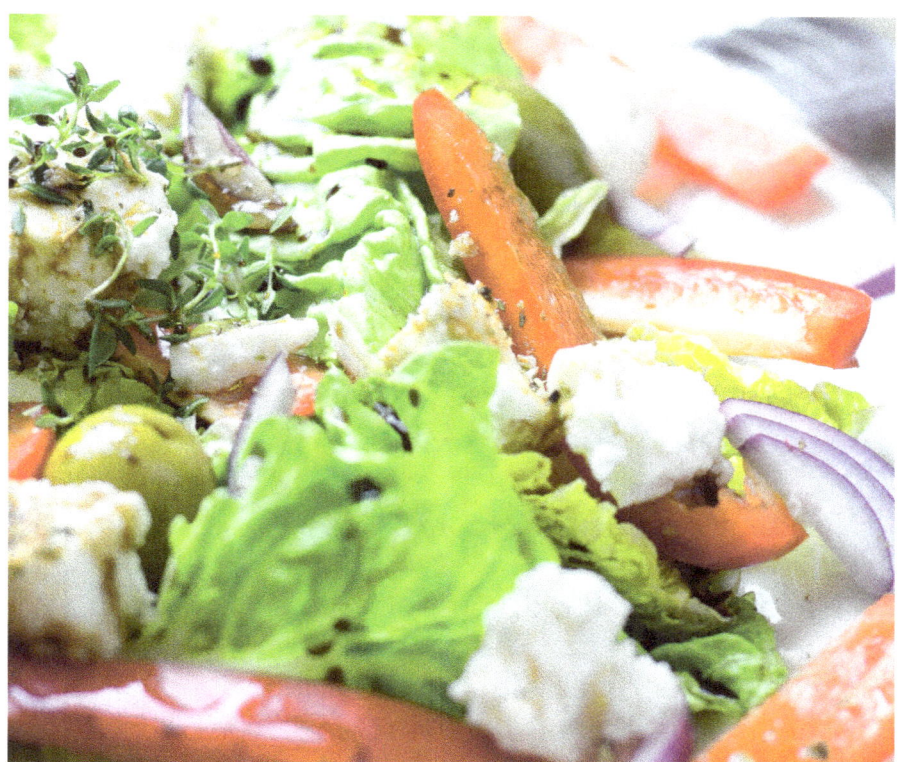

10. OKRA AND SPICED YOGURT

Cal.: 186 | Fat: 10.5g | Protein: 7.2g

Preparation Time: 8 minutes
Cooking Time: 75 hours
Servings: 6

Ingredients

2.5 lbs. fresh okra
4 tablespoons olive oil
1 ½ tablespoon lime zest
2 garlic cloves, crushed
Salt and white pepper, to taste

Yogurt:
1 cup Greek yogurt
2 teaspoons chili powder
¼ cup chopped cilantro

Directions

1. Preheat your cooker to 178°F/81°C.

2. Divide the fresh okra among two cooking bags.

3. Drizzle the okra with 2 ½ tablespoons olive oil (divided per bag), lime zest and season to taste.

Add one garlic clove per pouch.

4. Vacuum seal the bags and immerse in water.

5. Cook the okra for 1 hour. Remove from a water bath and drain the accumulated liquid in a bowl. Place the okra in a separate bowl.

6. In a medium bowl, combine Greek yogurt, chili powder, cilantro and accumulated okra water. Stir to combine.

7. Heat remaining vegetable oil during a skillet over medium-high heat.

8. Fry okra in the heated oil for 2 minutes.

9. Serve warm, with chili yogurt.

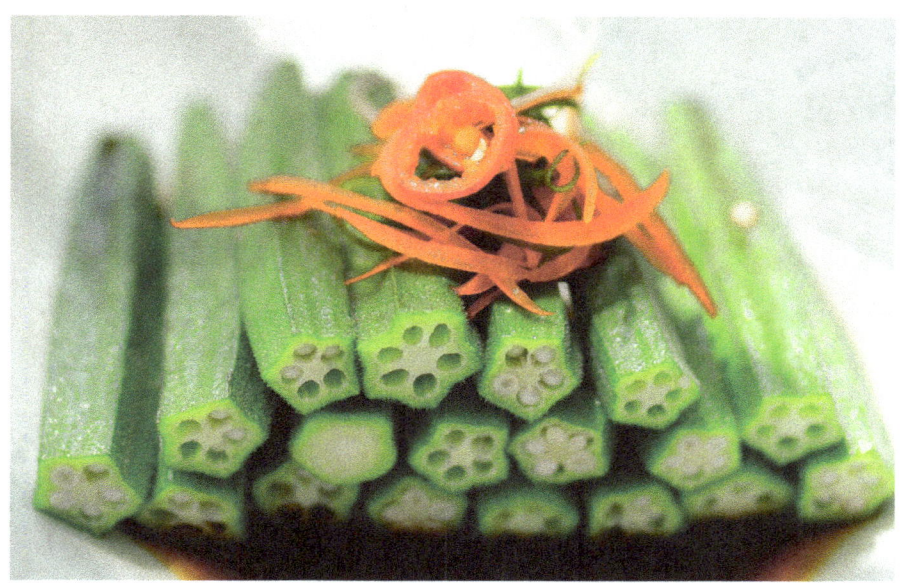

11. PARMESAN AND SCALLION OMELET

Cal.: 25 | Fat: 0.2g | Protein: 0.9g

Preparation Time: 6 minutes
Cooking Time: 30 minutes
Servings: 1

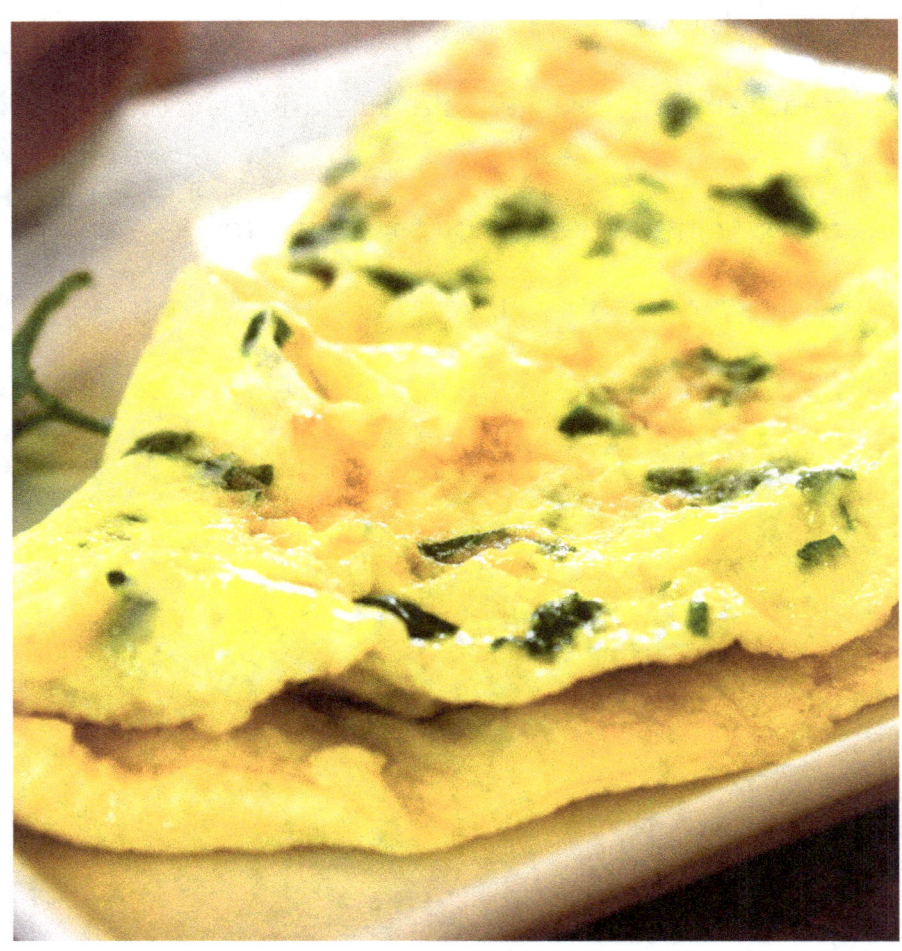

Ingredients

2 large eggs
1 tbsp. minced scallion greens
1 tbsp. finely grated Parmesan cheese
1 tbsp. unsalted butter, diced
Salt and pepper
Chopped fresh parsley, for serving

Directions

1. Preheat the Sous Vide machine to 165°F/73°C.

2. Whisk the eggs in a medium bowl. Then whisk in the parmesan, butter, scallions, and salt and pepper to taste.

3. Place the mixture in the bag that you're going to use to sous and seal it.

4. Place the bags in your preheated water and set the timer for 10 min.

5. After 10 minutes, gently fold the eggs into the shape of an omelet and cook for 10 more minutes.

6. Place the cooked omelet on a plate and top with the parsley to serve.

12. PERFECT EGG TOSTADA

Cal.: 354 | Fat: 28g | Protein: 16g

Preparation Time: 13 minutes
Cooking Time: 16 minutes
Servings: 4

Ingredients

4 large eggs, at room temperature
¼ cup cooked or canned black beans, heated
4 sprigs cilantro, chopped
4 corn tostadas
4 teaspoons salsa taquera or salsa Verde or chili de arbol
4 teaspoons Queso fresco, crumbled

Directions

1. Preheat the Sous Vide machine to 162°F/72°C. Place the eggs on a spoon, one at a time, and gently lower them into the water bath and place on the rack. Set the timer for 15 minutes. When the timer goes off, immediately remove the eggs from the water bath. Place the eggs in a bowl of cold water for a few minutes. To assemble: Place the tostadas on 4 serving plates. Spread a tablespoon of beans over it, then salsa, then sprinkle cheese on top and serve.

13. SOFT-POACHED EGGS

Cal.: 173 | Fat: 8.57g | Protein: 13.59g

Preparation Time: 2 minutes
Cooking Time: 12 minutes
Servings: 2

Ingredients

6 large eggs
2g Basil
A pinch of salt and pepper

Directions

1. Preheat a water bath to 75°C/167°F.

2. With a slotted spoon, lower the eggs into the bath. Be careful not to break them. Cook for 12 minutes straight, no more, no less.

3. In the meantime, grab a large bowl and fill it with water and ice. When the eggs are done, transfer them to an ice bowl. Let them cool for 2 minutes.

4. Serve with the salad of your choice or with keto toasts.

14. EGGS WITH ROASTED PEPPERS

Cal.: 144 | Fat: 10.7g | Protein: 9.4g

Preparation Time: 15 minutes
Cooking Time: 60 minutes
Servings: 6

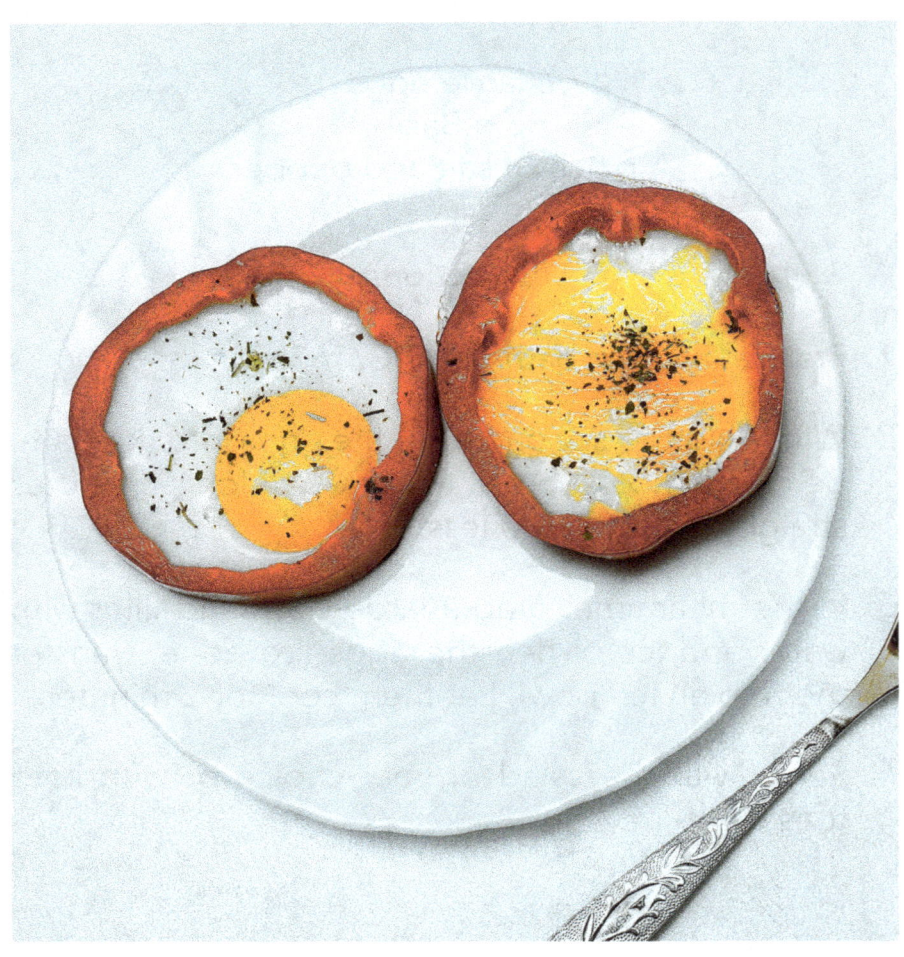

Ingredients

6 large eggs
½ cup grated Gouda cheese.
¼ cup cream cheese
3 roasted peppers (peeled and seeded)
Salt and pepper, to taste

Directions

1. Preheat the Sous Vide machine to 172°F/78°C.

2. In a food blender, blend eggs, Gouda cheese, cream cheese, salt and pepper.

3. Slice the peppers into thin strips.

4. Place the peppers in the bottom of six 4oz. jars, making sure they go up the sides a bit.

5. Pour the egg mixture. Attach two-part canning lids "fingertip tight."

6. Immerse in a water bath and cook for 1 hour.

7. Remove the jars from a water bath. Slide a knife around the peppers and eggs and remove carefully, or invert onto a plate.

8. Serve with warm bread.

15. EGG

Cal.: 274 | Fat: 21g | Protein: 15g

Preparation Time: 12 minutes
Cooking Time: 35 minutes
Servings: 1

Ingredients

1 egg
1 pinch of salt

Directions

1. Place the whole egg in a water bath heated to 144°F/62°C. Vacuum sealing is not necessary.

2. Cook the egg for 45 minutes. So, the yolk will be very runny. At 155°F/68°C, it becomes more solid.

3. Remove the egg from the water and rinse in cold water.

4. Whip up and place on a plate. Salt and pepper to taste.

16. ASPARAGUS WITH HOLLANDAISE

Cal.: 347 | Fat: 5.5g | Protein: 34.9g

Preparation Time: 21 minutes
Cooking Time: 30 minutes
Servings: 4

Ingredients

1 bunch asparagus, trimmed
Hollandaise

Directions

1. Preheat the water bath to 145°F/63°C. Place bagged sauce in the bath.

2. Set a timer for 30 minutes. When the timer has 12 minutes remaining, bag and seal asparagus.

3. Place in a water bath and cook for the remaining 10–12 minutes.

4. Remove cooked asparagus from the bath. Arrange on a plate. Blend sauce until smooth.

5. Pour over asparagus.

17. FLAX SEEDS MIX

Cal.: 230 | Fat: 12g | Protein: 13g

Preparation Time: 3 minutes
Cooking Time: 1 hour
Servings: 2

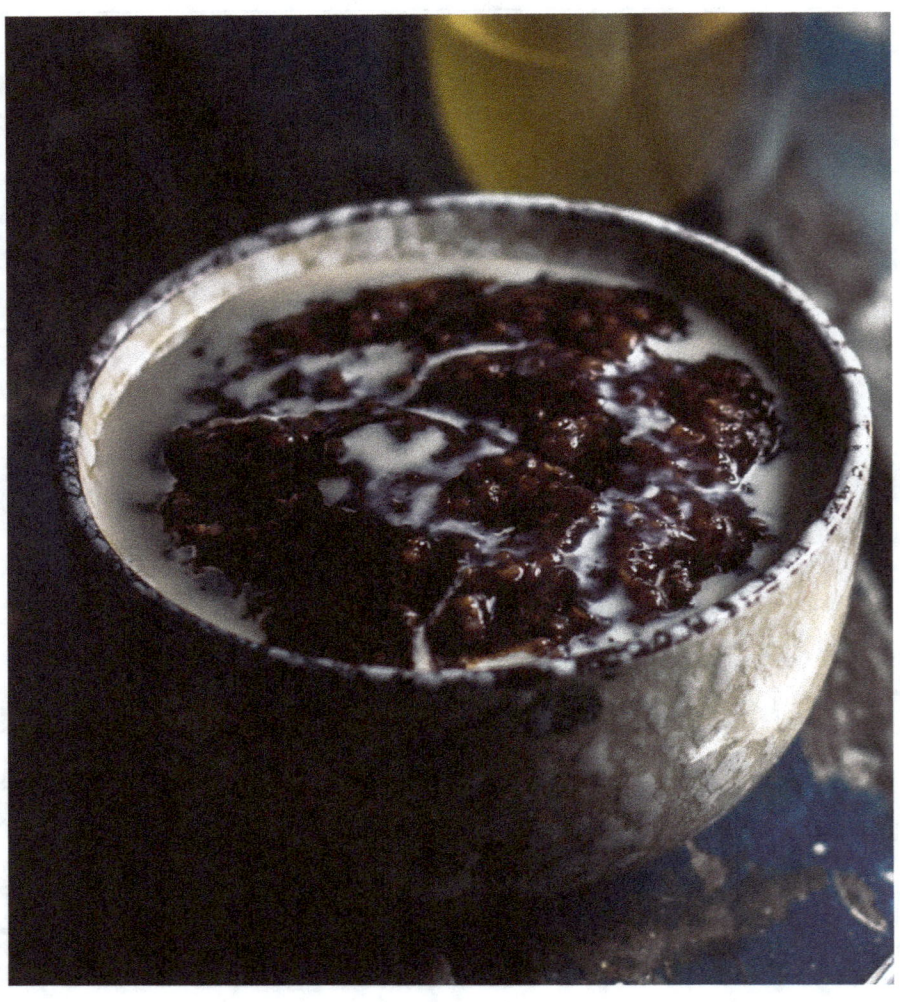

Ingredients

1/4 teaspoon stevia
2 tablespoons flax seeds
1 tablespoon sunflower seeds
1 cup almond milk
½ cup heavy cream
½ teaspoon cinnamon powder
¾ teaspoon vanilla extract

Directions

1. Prepare your sous-vide water bath to a temperature of 180°F/82°C.

2. Thoroughly mix the listed ingredients in a bowl.

3. Transfer the mixture to a Ziploc bag and seal the bag after squeezing out the excess air.

4. Lower the bag into the water bath and let it cook for 1 hour.

5. Once cooked, remove the bag from the water bath.

6. Transfer the porridge into serving bowls.

7. Serve and enjoy!

18. CIDER DIPPED FENNEL

Cal.: 67 | Fat: 0.4g | Protein: 2.2g

Preparation Time: 15 minutes
Cooking Time: 1 hour
Servings: 2

Ingredients

½ lb. fennel bulbs, chopped
Salt, to taste
2 tablespoons apple cider vinegar
Black pepper, to taste

Directions

1. Prepare and preheat the water bath at 190°F/88°C.

2. Add fennel and all the ingredients to a zipper-lock bag.

3. Seal the zipper-lock bag using the water immersion method. Place the sealed bag in the bath and cook for 1 hour.

4. Once done, transfer the fennel along with the sauce to a plate.

5. Serve.

19. CINNAMON AND EGG MIX

Cal.: 240 | Fat: 12g | Protein: 14g

Preparation Time: 10 minutes
Cooking Time: 30 minutes
Servings: 2

Ingredients

1/2 teaspoon Stevia sweetener
½ teaspoon cinnamon powder
1 teaspoon ginger powder
1/3 cup heavy cream
4 eggs, whisked

Directions

1. Prepare your sous-vide water bath to a temperature of 167°F/75°C.

2. Vacuum seal the entire ingredients in a cooking pouch. Lower the pouch into the preheated water bath and cook for 30 minutes.

3. Remove the pouch from the water bath and transfer the contents into serving bowls.

4. Serve and enjoy!

20. SIMPLE MUSHROOM SOUP

Cal.: 22 | Fat: 0.3g | Protein: 3.1g

Preparation Time: 4 minutes
Cooking Time: 40 minutes
Servings: 3

Ingredients

1 lb. mixed mushrooms
2 onions, diced
3 garlic cloves
2 sprigs parsley leaves, chopped
2 tbsp. thyme powder
2 tbsp. olive oil
2 cups cream
2 cups vegetable stock

Directions

1. Make a water bath, place a cooker in it, and set it at 185°F/85°C.

2. Place the mushrooms, onion and celery in a vacuum-sealable bag.

3. Release air by the water displacement method, seal and Immerse the bag in the water bath. Set the timer for 30 minutes. Once the timer has stopped,

remove and unseal the bag.

4. Blend the ingredients in the bag in a blender. Put a pan over medium heat, add the olive oil. Once it starts to heat, add the pureed mushrooms and the remaining listed ingredients except for the cream. Cook for 10 minutes.

5. Turn off heat and add cream. Stir well. Serve with a side of bread.

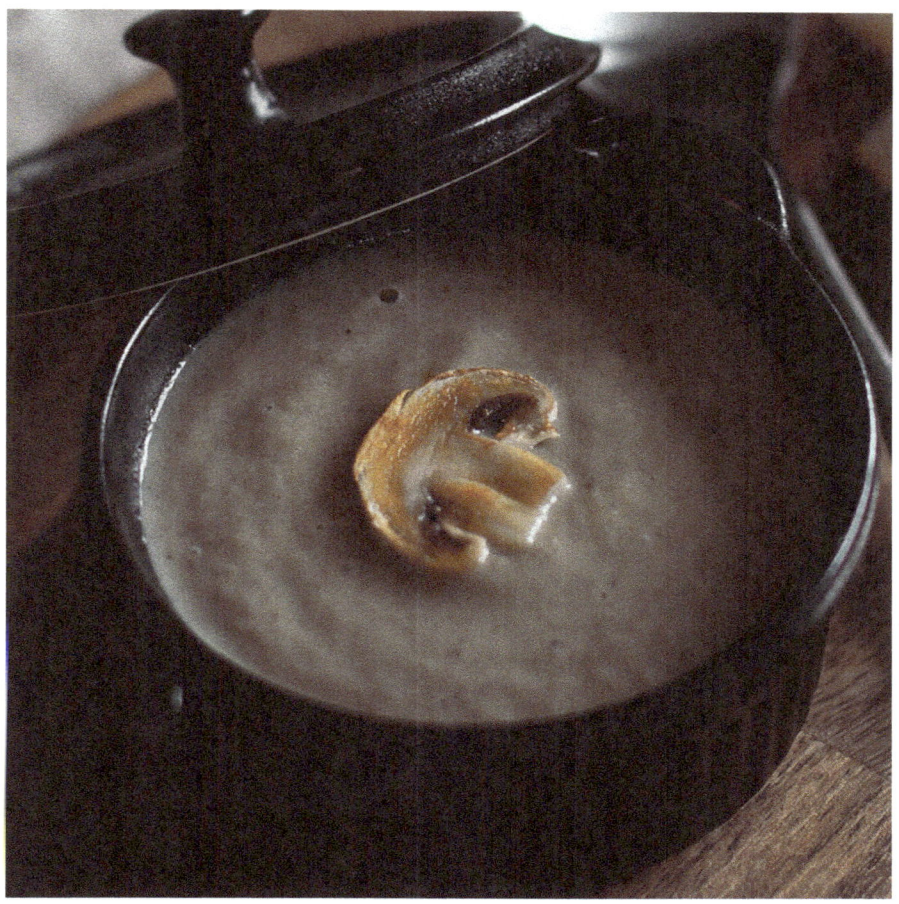

21. CAULIFLOWER SOUP

Cal.: 370 | Fat: 22g | Protein: 14g

Preparation Time: 9 minutes
Cooking Time: 70 minutes
Servings: 2

Ingredients

1 large head cauliflower, break into florets
2 shallots, chopped
4 cups of vegetable stock
½ cup white wine
½ cup sour cream
1 ½ cups cream
Juice of a lemon
1 teaspoon Ras el Hanout
Zest of 2 lemons, grated
A few slices of roasted caraway bread
1 teaspoon ground cumin
Cooking spray
1 cup grated cauliflower to serve
Extra virgin olive oil to serve

Directions

1. Place a skillet over medium heat. Spray with cooking spray. Add shallot and sauté for a couple of minutes.

2. Set your machine to 167°F/75°C. Place shallots, cauliflower, stock, and wine, sour cream, cream and lemon juice into a Ziploc or a vacuum-seal bag and remove all the air with the water displacement method or a vacuum-sealed. Seal and immerse the bag in the water bath.

3. Meanwhile mix together the grated cauliflower, Ras el Hanout and half of the lemon zest.

4. Remove the pouch from the cooker and transfer into the blender and blend until smooth. Season with salt and pepper. Pulse a couple of times to mix well.

5. Place the grated cauliflower mixture on bread slices. Drizzle some oil over it. Sprinkle salt, cumin and the remaining lemon zest.

6. Ladle into individual soup bowls. Serve with the garnished bread slices.

22. PORK CHOPS WITH MUSHROOMS

Cal.: 392 | Fat: 31.8g | Protein: 21g

Preparation Time: 10 minutes
Cooking Time: 2 hours 10 minutes
Servings: 4

Ingredients

4 pork chops, boneless
4 tbsp. butter
2 garlic cloves, minced
1 tbsp. flour
1 cup chicken broth
8 oz. cremini mushrooms, sliced
1 large shallot, sliced
Pepper
Salt

Directions

1. Preheat the Sous Vide machine to 140°F/60°C.

2. Place the chops into a Ziploc bag. Place the bag into a water bath and cook for 2 hours.

3. Remove the pork chops from the bag and pat dry with a paper towel.

4. Season the chop with salt and pepper.

5. Heat 2 tbsp. of butter in a pan. Sear the chops on both sides.

6. Add remaining 2 tbsp. of butter in a pan. Add sliced mushrooms to the pan and cook for 4–5 minutes stirring occasionally.

7. Add shallots, cook for 2 minutes until tender, add garlic and stir for 1 minute constantly, then add flour.

8. Stir well until mixture is evenly coated over mushrooms, add chicken broth, stir for 1 minute.

9. Season with salt and pepper. Serve and enjoy!

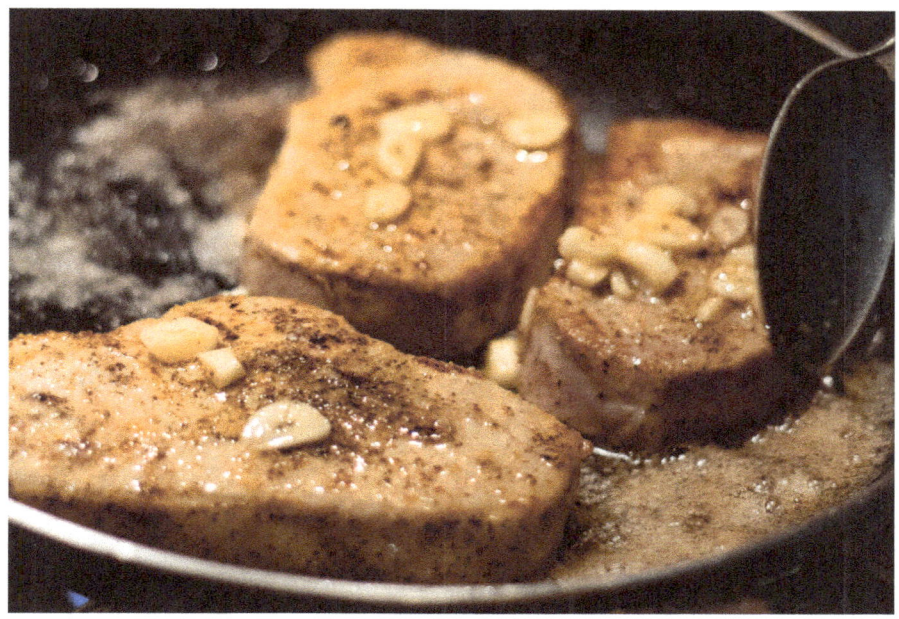

23. FAVORITE THAI DINNER

Cal.: 477 | Fat: 32.8g | Protein: 24.9g

Preparation Time: 14 minutes
Cooking Time: 76 minutes
Servings: 2

Ingredients

1 skinless, boneless chicken breast
Salt and freshly ground black pepper, to taste
2 tbsp. vegetable oil
½ cup cashews
2 cut into 1-inch segments scallions
2 tbsp. sweet chili sauce
1 tbsp. hoisin sauce
1 tsp. light soy sauces
1 tsp. chopped fresh cilantro

Directions

1. Fill and preheat the bath to 140°F/60°C.

2. Season the chicken breast with salt and pepper slightly.

3. In a cooking pouch, place the chicken breast.

4. Seal the pouch tightly after squeezing out the

excess air.

5. Place the pouches in the bath and cook for about 1¼ hours.

6. Remove the pouch from the bath.

7. Remove the chicken breast from the pouch and discard the cooking liquid.

8. Cut the chicken breast into bite-sized pieces.

9. In a skillet, heat the oil on medium heat and stir fry the cashews and scallions for about 2 minutes.

10. Stir in all sauces and chicken breast; and fry for about 1 minute.

11. Serve hot with the garnishing of cilantro.

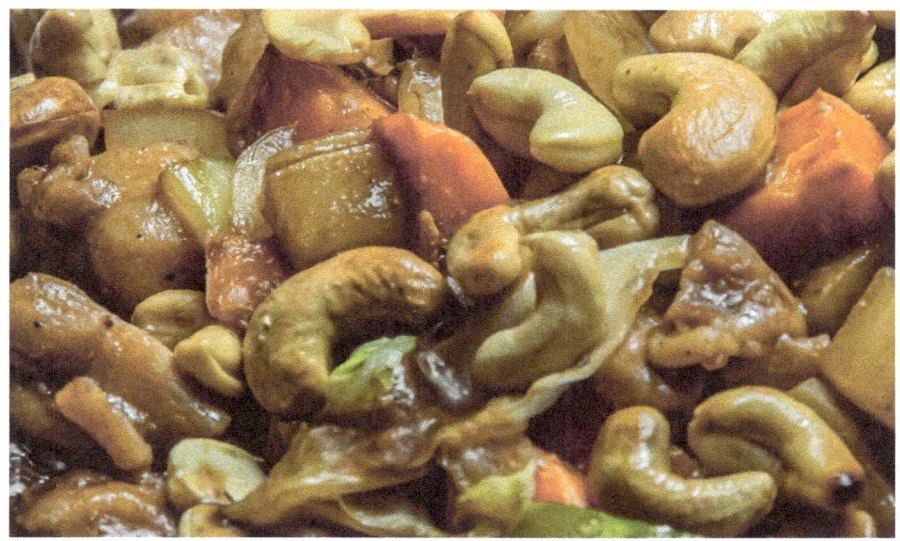

24. MID-WEEK CHICKEN

Cal.: 146 | Fat: 6g | Protein: 16g

Preparation Time: 11 minutes
Cooking Time: 30 minutes
Servings: 4

Ingredients

4 (6-ounce) skinless, boneless chicken breasts
Salt and freshly ground black pepper, to taste
3 tbsp. butter
1 sliced crosswise large leek
½ cup panko breadcrumbs
1-ounce shredded sharp cheddar cheese
2 tbsp. chopped fresh parsley
1 tbsp. olive oil

Directions

1. Fill and preheat the bath to 145°F/63°C.

2. Season the chicken breasts with salt and pepper evenly. In a cooking pouch, place the chicken breasts.

3. Seal the pouch tightly after squeezing out the excess air.

4. Place the pouch in the bath and cook for about 45 minutes.

5. Meanwhile, in a skillet, melt 2 tbsp. of butter on medium heat.

6. Stir in leeks, salt and black pepper. Reduce heat to low and cook for about 10 minutes.

7. Remove from the heat and keep aside. In a frying pan, melt the remaining butter on medium heat.

8. Add the panko and toast till golden, stirring continuously.

9. Transfer the toasted panko in a bowl with cheddar and parsley and toss to coat well. Remove the pouch from the bath.

10. Remove the chicken breasts from the pouch and discard the cooking liquid. With paper towels, gently pat dry the chicken breasts.

11. In a skillet, heat olive oil on high heat and sear the chicken breasts for about 1 minute per side.

12. Divide the cooked leek into serving plates and top each with 1 chicken breast.

13. Sprinkle with toasted panko mixture and serve immediately.

25. PORK TENDERLOIN

Cal.: 440 | Fat: 20.7g | Protein: 59g

Preparation Time: 16 minutes
Cooking Time: 2 hours
Servings: 4

Ingredients

16 oz. pork tenderloin
1 tbsp. olive oil
1 tbsp. butter
2 small shallots, sliced
2 garlic cloves
8 sprigs of fresh herbs
Black pepper
Kosher salt

Directions

1. Preheat the Sous Vide machine to 150 °F/66°C.

2. Season the pork with salt and pepper.

3. Place the pork into a Ziploc bag. Remove all the air from the bag before sealing.

4. Place the bag into the hot water bath and cook for 2 hours.

5. Remove pork from the Ziploc bag and pat dry with a paper towel.

6. Heat olive oil in a pan over medium heat. Add pork and cook for 2 minutes until lightly browned.

7. Add butter with fresh thyme, shallots, and garlic. Cook for 1 minute.

8. Serve and enjoy!

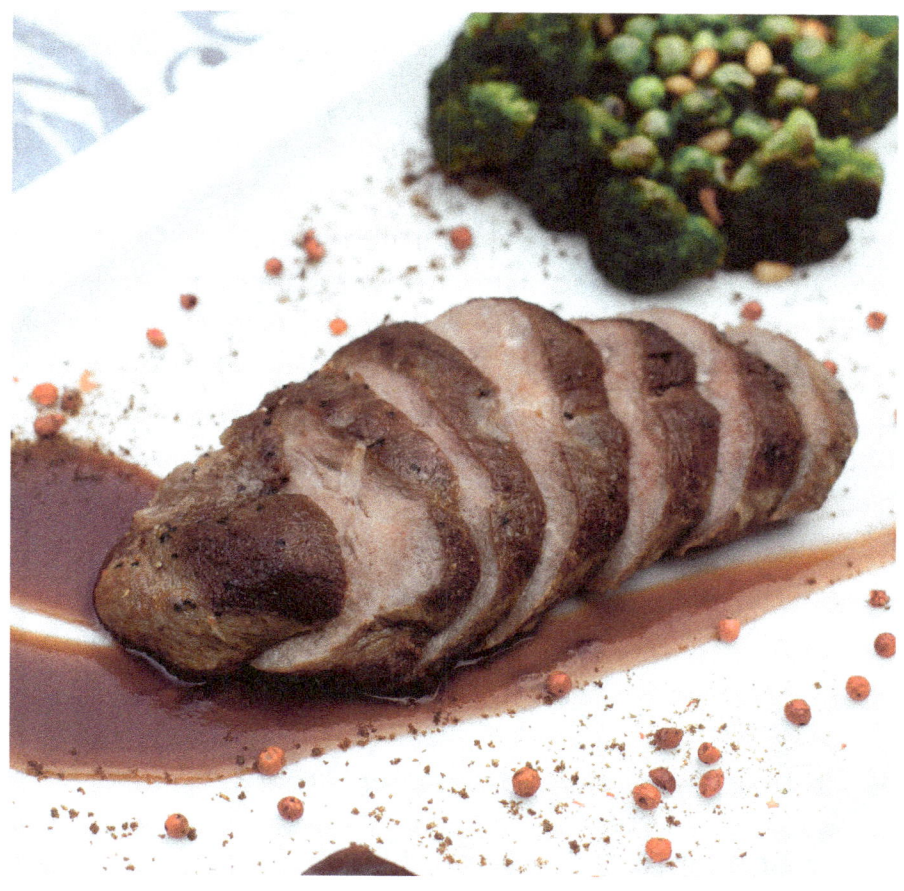

26. LAMB CHOPS WITH BASIL CHIMICHURRI

Cal.: 435 | Fat: 44.8g | Protein: 8.4g

Preparation Time: 10 minutes
Cooking Time: 2 hours
Servings: 4

Ingredients

2 rack of lamb, drenched
2 garlic cloves, crushed
Pepper
Salt
For basil Chimichurri:
3 tbsp. red wine vinegar
½ cup olive oil
1 tsp. red chili flakes
2 garlic cloves, minced
1 shallot, diced
1 cup fresh basil, chopped
1/4 tsp. pepper
1/4 tsp. sea salt

Directions

1. Preheat the Sous Vide machine to 132°F/56°C.

2. Season lamb with pepper and salt.

3. Place lamb in a large Ziploc bag with garlic and remove all air from the bag before sealing.

4. Place the bag into the hot water bath and cook for 2 hours.

5. Add all chimichurri ingredients to the bowl and mix well. Place in the refrigerator for minutes.

6. Remove lamb from the bag and pat dry with a paper towel.

7. Sear lamb in hot oil. Slice lamb between the bones.

8. Place seared lamb chops on a serving dish and top with chimichurri. Serve and enjoy!

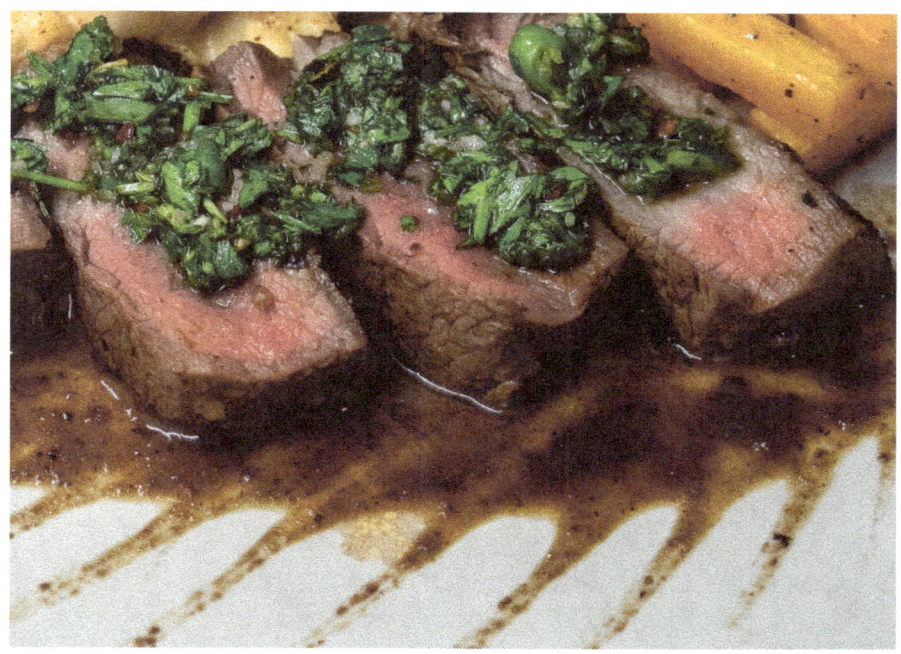

27. CHIPOTLE APPLE PORK LOIN

Cal.: 548 | Fat: 34g | Protein: 51g

Preparation Time: 11 minutes
Cooking Time: 4 hours
Servings: 6

Ingredients

1 tsp. salt
1 tsp. black pepper
½ tsp. pork loin chipotle powder
¼ tsp. ground cloves
¼ tsp. ground nutmeg
2 lbs. pork loin
2 tbsp. apple concentrate
1 tbsp. maple syrup
1 tbsp. coconut oil

Directions

1. Preheat the Sous Vide machine to 134°F /56.7°C.

2. Place the rub ingredients in a bowl and mix them together.

3. Coat the pork with the rub mixture.

4. Place the pork in the bag you're going to use to sous, pour in the apple concentrate, maple syrup and coconut oil, and seal the bag.

5. Place the bag in the preheated water and set the timer for 4 hours.

6. When the pork is done allow it to rest for 5 minutes.

7. Slice and serve the pork.

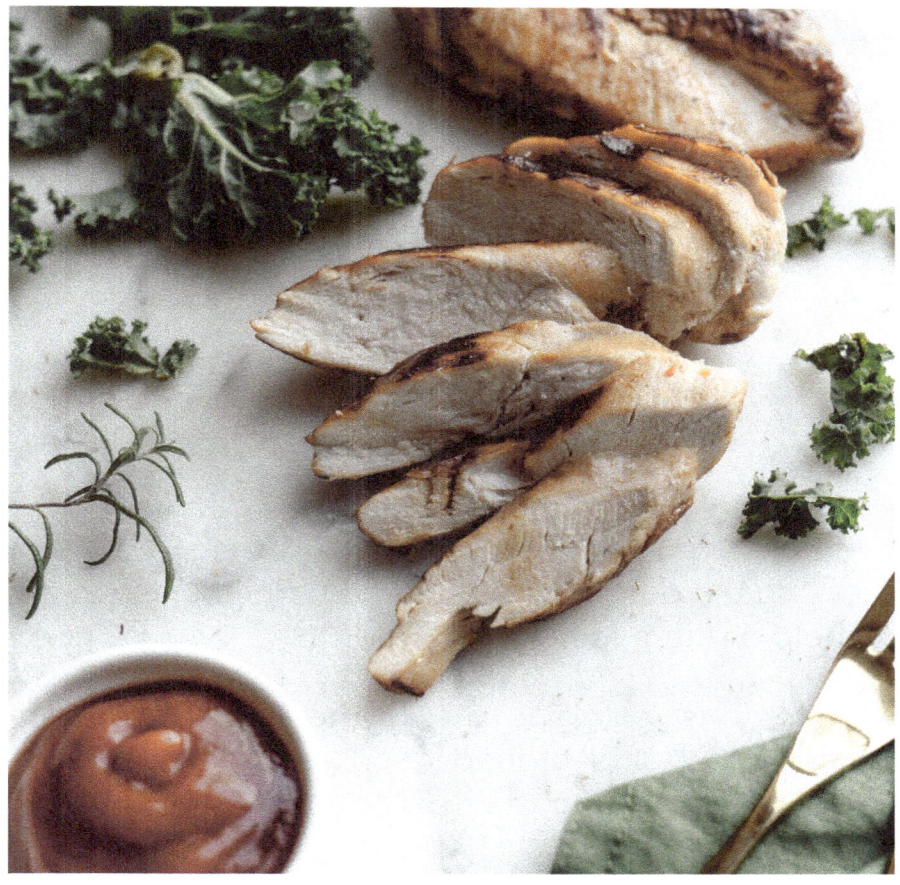

28. FRENCH DUCK CONFIT

Cal.: 272 | Fat: 15.3g | Protein: 30g

Preparation Time: 20 minutes
Cooking Time: 15 hours
Servings: 4

Ingredients

16 oz. duck legs
1 teaspoon thyme
1 teaspoon coriander
1 teaspoon lime zest
2 tablespoon kaffir leaves
A pinch of Stevia sweetener
1 teaspoon salt
1 tablespoon orange peel
1 teaspoon ground paprika
2 teaspoon sesame oil

Directions

1. Wash the duck legs carefully and dry them with the help of the paper towel.

2. After this, combine the thyme, coriander, palm stevia, salt and ground paprika together. Stir the spices gently with the help of the fork.

3. After this, wash the kaffir leaves and place them in the blender.

4. Add the kaffir leaves and orange peel.

5. Blend the mixture until it is smooth.

6. Transfer the dried duck legs in the plastic bag.

7. Then add the mixed spices and blended lemon zest mixture.

8. Close the plastic bag and shake it well.

9. After this, seal the plastic bag.

10. Set the water bath to 160°F/71°C and place the sealed plastic bag with the duck legs there.

11. Cook the dish for 15 hours. After this time, you will get totally tender duck legs.

12. When the time is over, transfer the duck legs in the serving plates or use one serving plate for everyone.

13. Serve it!

29. SAUSAGE TOMATO

Cal.: 250 | Fat: 12g | Protein: 18g

Preparation Time: 9 minutes
Cooking Time: 43 minutes
Servings: 4

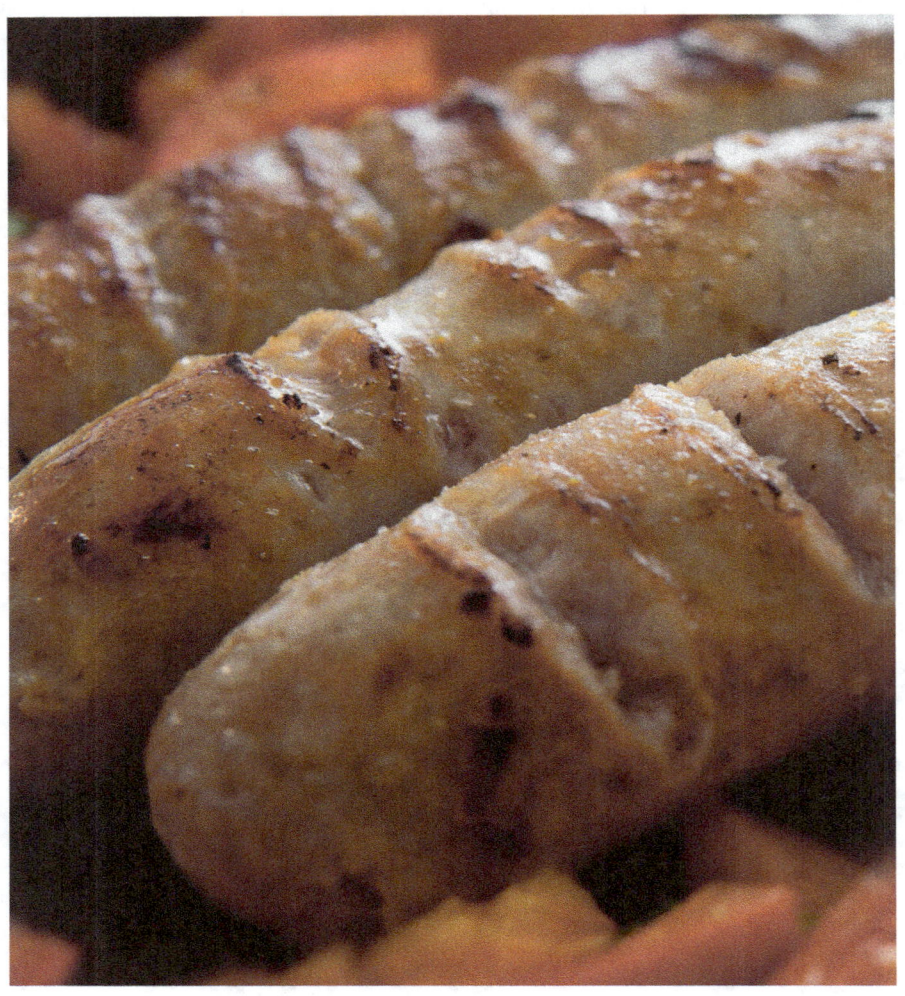

Ingredients

1 cup baby spinach
1 tablespoon avocado oil
2 pork sausage links, sliced
1 cup cherry tomatoes, halved
1 cup kalamata olives, pitted and halved
2 tablespoons lemon juice
2 tablespoons basil pesto
Salt and black pepper to the taste

Directions

1. Prepare your sous vide water bath to a temperature of 180°F/82°C.

2. Get a cooking pouch and add all the listed ingredients.

3. Immerse the pouch into the water bath and let it cook for 40 minutes.

4. Once done, remove the pouch from the water bath.

5. Transfer the contents into two serving bowls.

6. Serve and enjoy!

30. SPICE RUBBED SHORT RIBS

Cal.: 428 | Fat: 26.1g | Protein: 67g

Preparation Time: 11 minutes
Cooking Time: 48 hours
Servings: 6

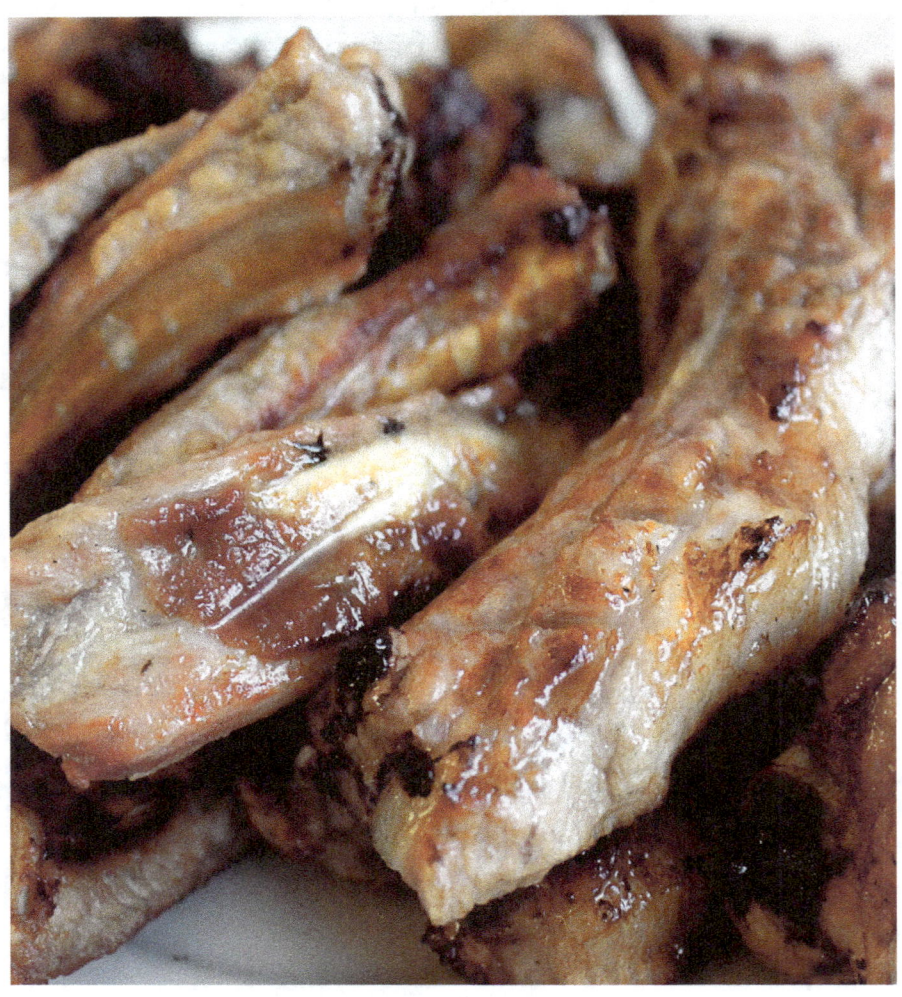

Ingredients

1 tbsp. ground cumin
1 tbsp. ancho chili powder
1/4 tsp. ground cloves
1 tsp. Kosher salt
1 tsp. freshly ground black pepper
3 lbs. beef short ribs

Directions

1. Preheat the Sous Vide machine to 140°F/60°C.

2. Combine the spices in a bowl. Coat the beef ribs with the spice rub.

3. Place the steak in the bag or bags you're going to use to sous and seal the bag or bags.

4. Place the bag in your preheated water and set the timer for 48 hours.

5. When the ribs are almost ready, preheat your broiler.

6. Place the cooked ribs on an aluminum foil-rimmed baking sheet or pan. Broil for about 5 minutes, until you see the edges char.

7. Serve immediately.

31. MISO SOY GLAZED PORK CHOPS

Cal.: 568 | Fat: 36.1g | Protein: 57g

Preparation Time: 75 minutes
Cooking Time: 1 hour
Servings: 2

Ingredients

4 whole pork chops, bone-in
1/3 cup mirin japanese cooking wine
1/3 cup low sodium soy sauce
2 tbsp. white miso paste
2 garlic cloves, minced
1/2 teaspoon Stevia sweetener
2 tbsp. butter, cubed
Green onion, chopped (garnish)
Sesame seeds, for garnish

Directions

1. Place the mirin, miso, soy sauce, stevia and garlic in a bowl. Use a whisk to mix the ingredients until the miso and stevia dissolve.

2. Divide the pork chops between 2 large resealable plastic bags. Pour in half the sauce to each bag. Place the sealed bag in your refrigerator for at least

1 hour. Then preheat the Sous Vide machine to 140°F /60°C.

3. Remove the air from the plastic bags and place them in your preheated water.

4. Set the timer for 1 hour.

5. While the pork chops are cooking, preheat a grill to high heat.

6. Use a paper towel to pat the cooked pork chops dry. Put the sauce from the bag in a saucepan.

7. Bring the sauce to a simmer. Once simmering, cook for 8 to 10 minutes.

8. Then use a whisk to mix in the butter. Remove the pan from the heat.

9. Put the pork chops on the preheated grill. Sear the pork chops for about 1 to 2 minutes per side.

10. Top the seared pork chops with the thicken sauce and top with green onions and sesame seeds to serve.

32. INDIAN STYLE PORK

Cal.: 363 | Fat: 12.7g | Protein: 19.5g

Preparation Time: 15 minutes
Cooking Time: 2 hours
Servings: 4

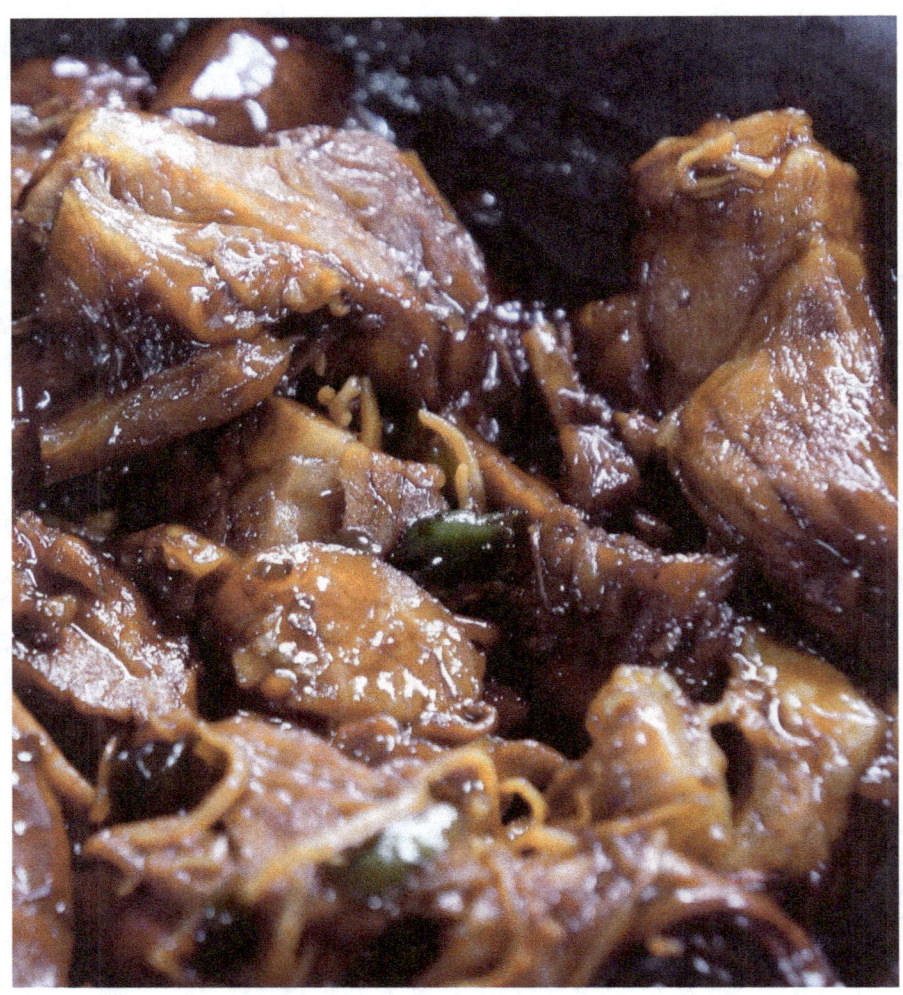

Ingredients

1.5lb. Pork tenderloin, sliced
2 cups yogurt
1 cup sour cream
2 tablespoons tandoori paste
1 tablespoon curry paste
1-inch ginger, minced
2 garlic cloves, minced
Salt and pepper, to taste

Directions

1. In a large bowl, combine yogurt, sour cream, tandoori paste, curry paste, garlic, and ginger. Add sliced pork.

2. Cover and marinate for 20 minutes in a fridge. Preheat your cooker to 135°F/57°C.

3. Remove the pork from the marinade and place into the bag. Vacuum seal the bag. Immerse pork in the water bath and cook for 2 hours.

4. Remove the bag from water and open carefully. Heat 1 tablespoon olive oil in a large skillet. Sear the pork for 3 minutes per side. Serve warm.

33. WARM BEEF SOUP WITH GINGER

Cal.: 214 | Fat: 35g | Protein: 1g

Preparation Time: 15 minutes
Cooking Time: 4 hours
Servings: 8

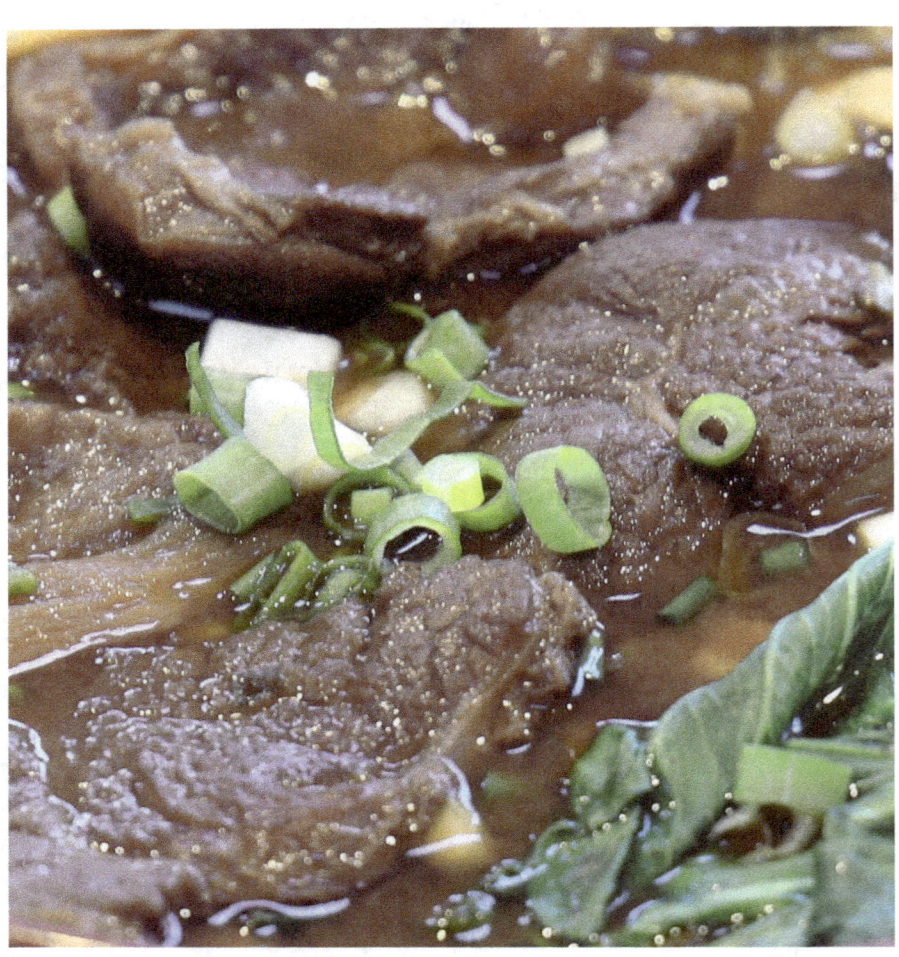

Ingredients

2 lbs. chopped beef
¼ cup chopped onion
½ cup chopped celery
¼ tsp. pepper
½ tsp. nutmeg
½ tsp. ginger
2 quarts water

Directions

1. Preheat an oven to 450°F/232° then line a baking sheet with parchment paper. Set aside.

2. Place the beef in a bowl together with chopped onion, celery, pepper, nutmeg and ginger. Mix well.

3. Place all on the prepared baking sheet and bake for about 10 minutes.

4. Meanwhile, preheat the Sous Vide machine to 145°F/63°C and wait until it reaches the targeted temperature.

5. Next, remove the beef from the oven and transfer all to a big plastic bag. Pour water into the bag then seal it properly and cook for 4 hours.

6. Once it is done, transfer to a serving bowl and enjoy immediately.

34. PERFECTLY COOKED MUSHROOMS

Cal.: 94 | Fat: 3.22g | Protein: 5.02g

Preparation Time: 11 minutes
Cooking Time: 30 minutes
Servings: 4

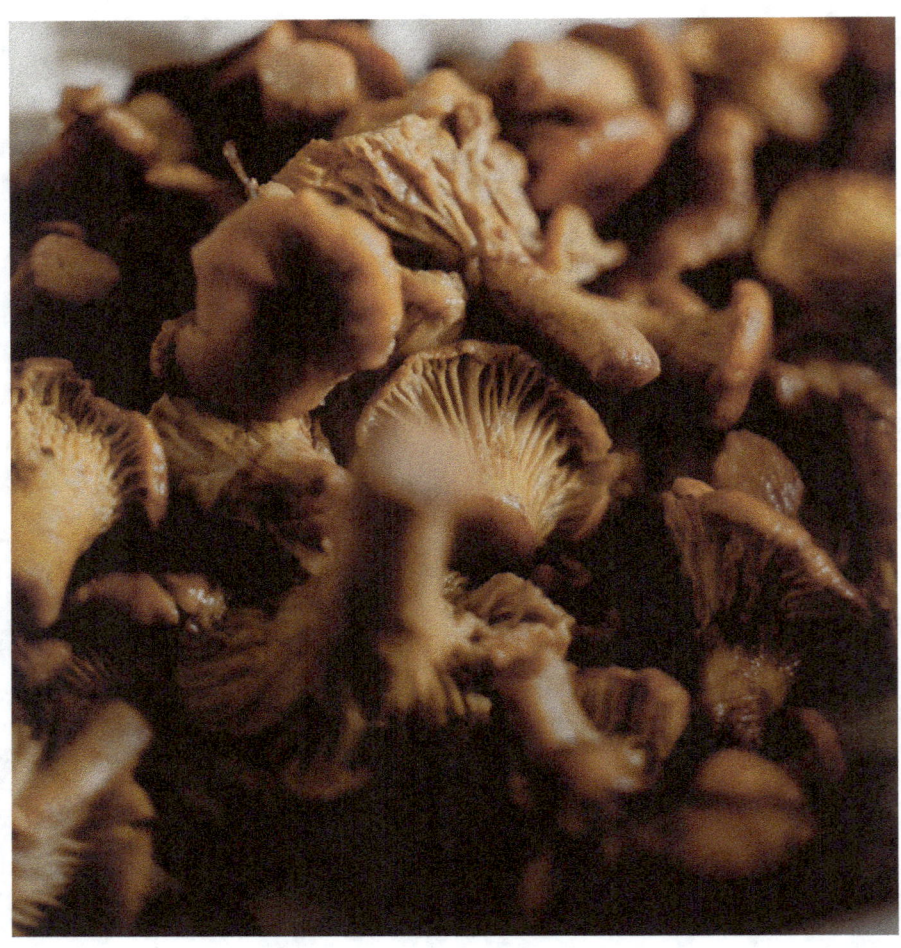

Ingredients

450g/1lb. mixed mushrooms, thoroughly washed and cut into tiny pieces
2 tbsp./1Fl.oz. Extra-virgin olive oil
2 tsp. fresh thyme leaves
1 tbsp./0.5Fl.oz. Balsamic vinegar
2 tbsp./1Fl.oz. Soy sauce
½ tsp. black pepper
Salt to taste

Directions

1. Preheat a water bath to 80°C/176°F.

2. In the meanwhile, add mushrooms and all ingredients to a big bowl. Stir thoroughly so that the ingredients cover mushrooms.

3. Place the mixture in the plastic bag and seal.

4. Let it cook for 30 minutes.

5. When done, remove the bag from the bath.

6. Serve warm.

35. TENDER LEEKS WITH HERBED BUTTER

Cal.: 130 | Fat: 11.7g | Protein: 0.8g

Preparation Time: 11 minutes
Cooking Time: 1 hour
Servings: 4

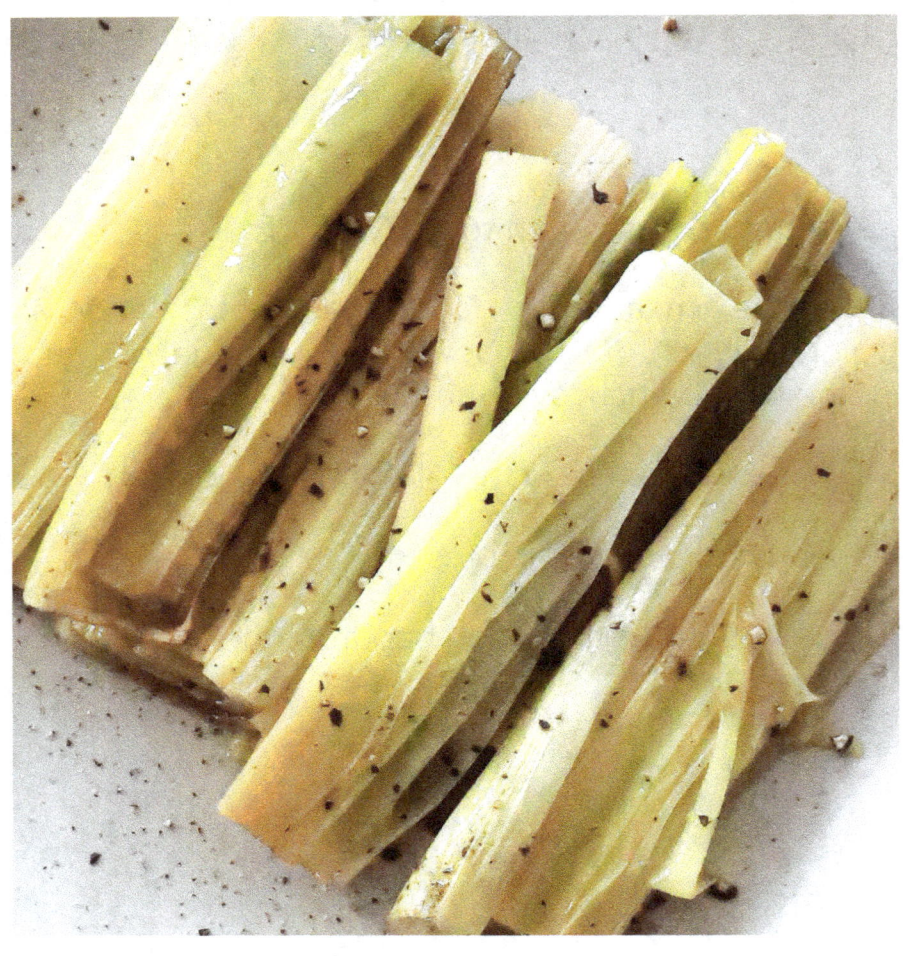

Ingredients

4 baby leeks (or 2 large)
4 tablespoons butter, salted
1 teaspoon Herbes de Provence

Directions

1. Preheat the Sous Vide machine to 180°F/82°C.

2. Wash leeks and cut off ends. If using large leeks, split down the middle, then cut again in half, making four sections per leek. Baby leeks can be left intact.

3. Melt butter in the microwave, add herbs, and mix.

4. Put leeks and butter into a large zipper-lock bag, swirl the butter mixture around to evenly coat the leeks. Remove excess air and seal shut.

5. Place in the bath and cook for one hour.

6. Serve as a tender side dish for any main course.

36. PARMESAN GARLIC ASPARAGUS

Cal.: 85 | Fat: 1g | Protein: 0.9g

Preparation Time: 6 minutes
Cooking Time: 16 minutes
Servings: 4

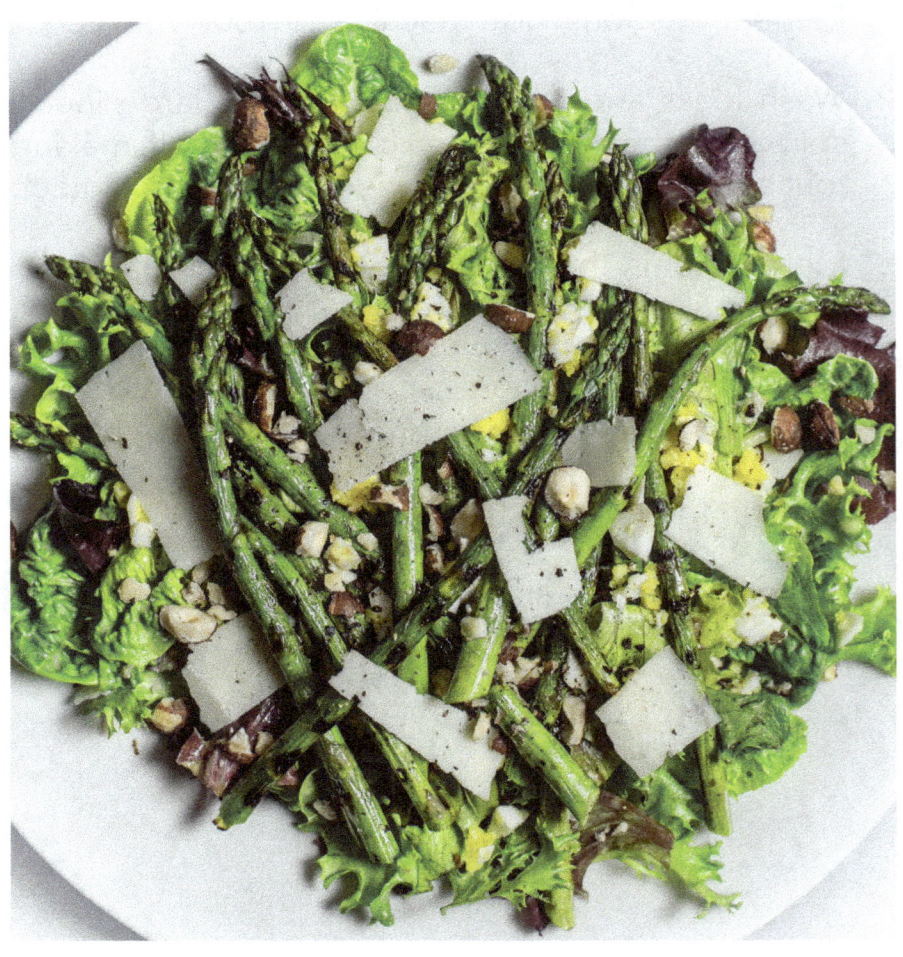

Ingredients

1 bunch green asparagus, trimmed
4 tbsp. unsalted butter, cut into cubes
Sea salt
1 tbsp. pressed garlic
1/4 cup shaved Parmesan cheese

Directions

1. Preheat the Sous Vide machine to 185°F/85°C.

2. Use paper towels to pat the salmon dry

3. Place the asparagus in a single layer row in the bag or bags you're going to use to sous. Put a tbsp. butter in each of the corners, the pressed garlic in the middle, salt to taste, and seal the bag. Move the bag around to get garlic to disperse evenly.

4. Place the bag in your preheated water and set the timer for 14 minutes.

5. Top the cooked asparagus with some of the liquid from the bag and the parmesan cheese.

6. Serve immediately.

37. CHILI AND GARLIC SAUCE

Cal.: 25 | Fat: 0.2g | Protein: 0.9g

Preparation Time: 7 minutes
Cooking Time: 30 minutes
Servings: 15

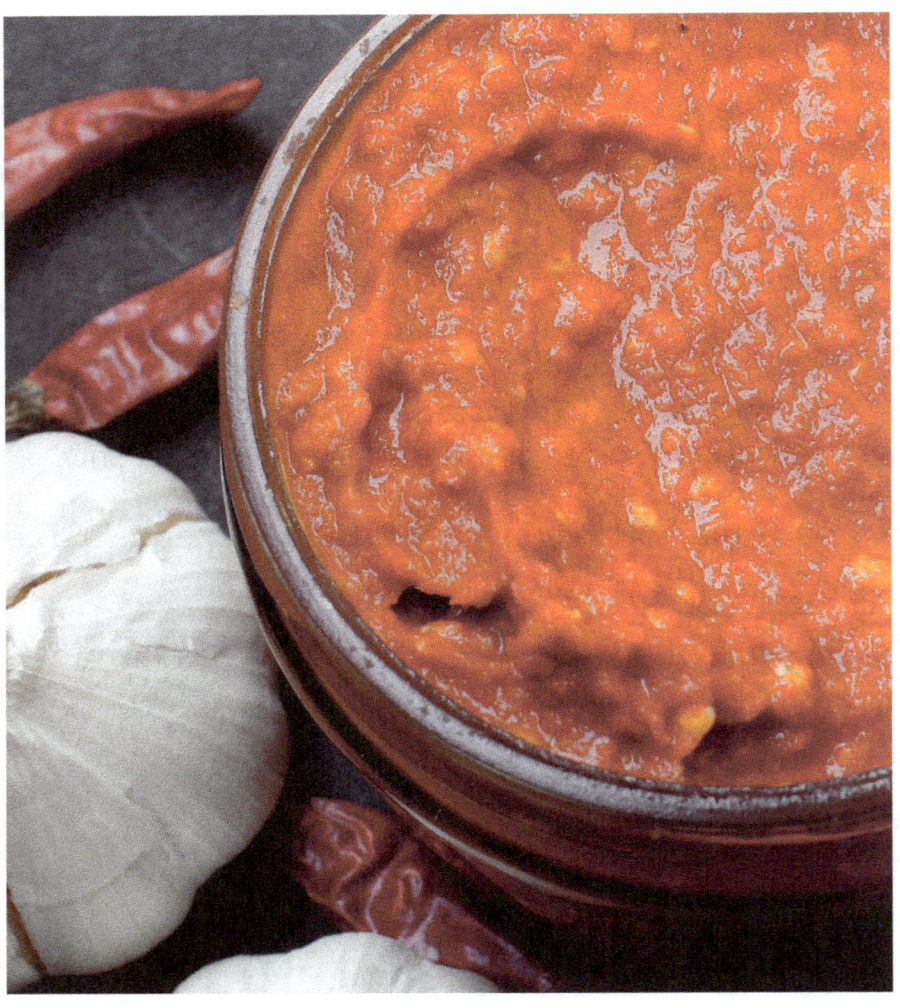

Ingredients

2 lb. red chili peppers
4 garlic cloves, crushed
2 tsp. smoked paprika
1 cup cilantro leaves, chopped
½ cup basil leaves, chopped
2 lemons' juice

Directions

1. Make a water bath, place a cooker in it, and set it at 185°F/85°C.

2. Place the peppers in a vacuum-sealable bag.

3. Release air by the water displacement method, seal and Immerse the bag in the water bath. Set the timer for 30 minutes.

4. Once the timer has stopped, remove and unseal the bag.

5. Transfer the pepper and the remaining listed ingredients to a blender and purée to smooth.

6. Store in an airtight container, refrigerate and use for up to 7 days.

38. TURMERIC PICKLED CAULIFLOWER

Cal.: 125 | Fat: 21g | Protein: 11g

Preparation Time: 11 minutes
Cooking Time: 3 hours
Servings: 6

Ingredients

4 cups Cauliflower Florets
1 cup White Wine Vinegar
1 cup Water
1/4 teaspoon Stevia sweetener
1 tbsp. Salt
1 Thumb-Sized Piece Turmeric sliced
A few Sprigs Dill
1 tbsp. Black Peppercorns

Directions

1. Preheat the Sous Vide machine to 140°F/60°C.

2. Place everything but the dill and cauliflower in a small pot and bring to a simmer on medium heat. Stir the mixture carefully until the stevia dissolves.

3. Place the cauliflower and dill in the bag you're going to use to sous along with the heated mixture

and seal the bag.

4. Place the bag in your preheated water and set the timer for 3 hours.

5. Towards the end of the cooking process, prepare an ice bath, which is half ice half water.

6. Place the cooked cauliflower, still in the bag in the ice bath and let it chill for 15 minutes before serving.

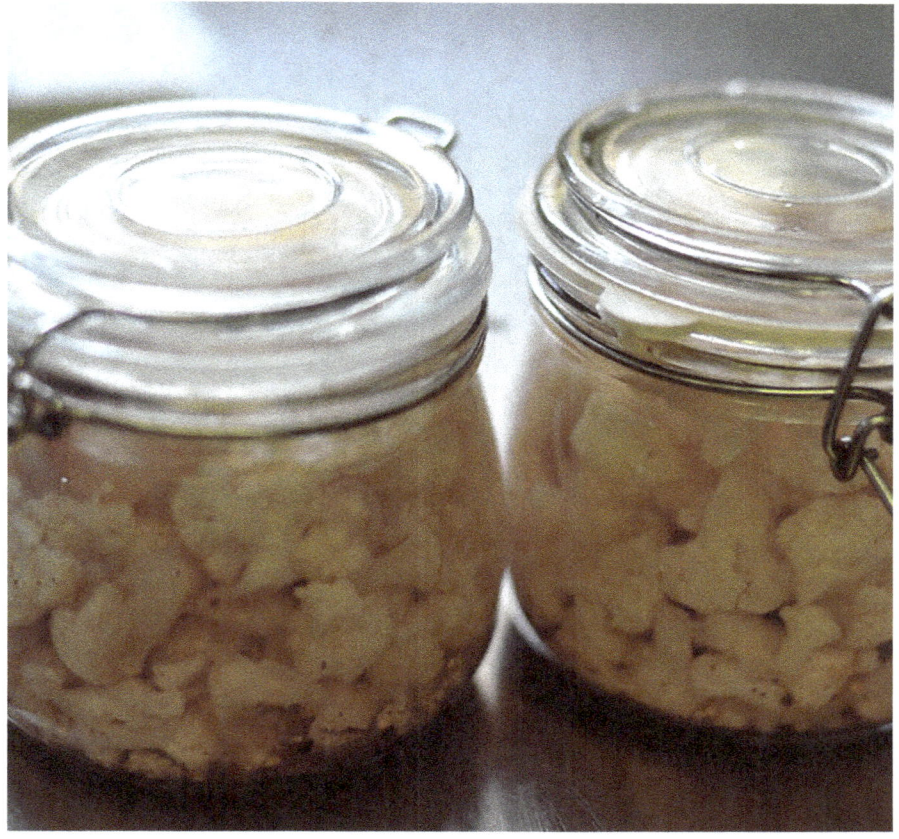

Photo: "pickled cauliflower" by manthatcooks

39. GARLIC DIPPING SAUCE WITH ASPARAGUS

Cal.: 232 | Fat: 15g | Protein: 2g

Preparation Time: 12 minutes
Cooking Time: 40 minutes
Servings: 8

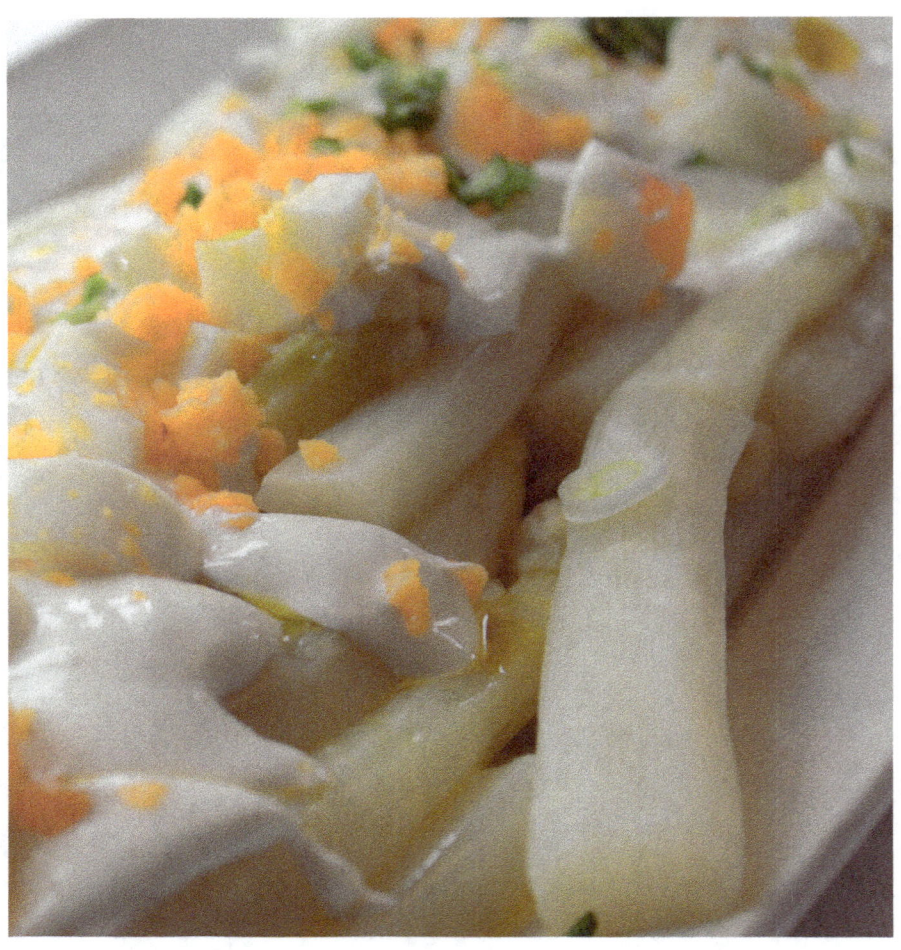

Ingredients

½ stick butter, melted
Sea salt and black pepper, to taste
1 ½ pounds asparagus spears, halved lengthwise
4 garlic cloves, minced
1/4 cup sour cream
10 garlic cloves, smashed
Salt and pepper, to taste
1/4 cup mayonnaise
½ cup plain yogurt

Directions

1. Prepare your sous-vide water bath to a temperature of 183°F/84°C.

2. In a Ziploc bag, put the asparagus spears, black pepper, butter, garlic cloves and salt into and seal it after squeezing out the excess air.

3. Lower the pouch in the water bath and cook for 30 minutes.

4. For the dipping, get a bowl and thoroughly mix all the remaining ingredients.

5. Serve asparagus with dipping sauce.

40. SCALLOPS WITH LEMON HERB SALSA VERDE

Cal.: 459 | Fat: 34g | Protein: 16g

Preparation Time: 15 minutes
Cooking Time: 60 minutes
Servings: 2

Ingredients

8 Sea scallops, side muscle removed
Pink Himalayan salt and pepper, to taste
1 tbsp. olive oil
1 tbsp. ghee or butter
¼ cup fresh cilantro, parsley, chives and basil, roughly chopped
Juice from ½ Lemon
¼ cup olive oil
1 small shallot, minced
1 garlic clove, minced

Directions

1. Preheat the water bath to 123.8°F/51°C.

2. Salt and pepper scallops on both sides and place in a Ziploc bag in a single layer.

3. Pour in 1 tbsp. olive oil.

4. Place the scallops into your water bath using the water displacement method.

5. Cook for 30 minutes.

6. While scallops are cooking, prepare your salsa Verde.

7. Add your chopped herbs into a bowl with the shallot, garlic and lemon juice and stir to combine.

8. Let sit for 5 minutes and then mix in the ¼ cup olive oil and set aside.

9. When the scallops are finished cooking, remove from the water bath

10. Remove them from the bag and carefully place them on a plate and pat dry.

11. Heat the ghee/butter on high heat in a cast-iron skillet.

12. When the ghee is melted, add the Scallops, one at a time and cook for 45 seconds on each side.

13. Serve with salsa Verde.

41. SWORDFISH WITH BALSAMIC BROWN BUTTER SAUCE

Cal.: 634 | Fat: 34.5g | Protein: 64.3g

Preparation Time: 21 minutes
Cooking Time: 34 minutes
Servings: 4

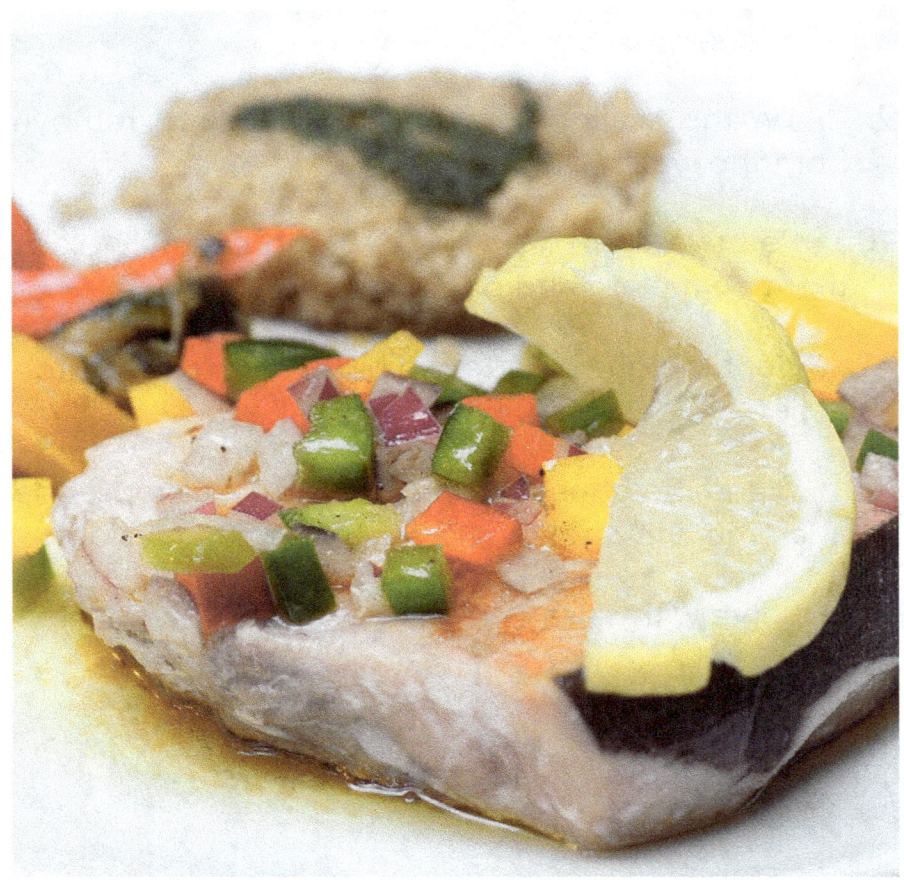

Ingredients

2 lbs. swordfish steaks
Salt and pepper
Zest from ½ lemon
1 stick unsalted butter
3 tbsp. balsamic vinegar
3 tbsp. honey
1 tablespoon Dijon mustard

Directions

1. Preheat the Sous Vide machine to 126°F/52°C.

2. Salt and pepper your steaks to taste and season with lemon zest.

3. Place the steaks in the bag and place in the water bath for 30 minutes.

4. Add the butter in a saucepan over medium heat until it foams. Once it stops foaming and turns a golden brown, whisk in the balsamic vinegar, Dijon and honey. Lower the heat to a simmer and allow the sauce to thicken.

5. Remove the steaks from the bag and top with the sauce to serve.

42. SAVORY HALIBUT

Cal.: 341 | Fat: 26.9g | Protein: 22g

Preparation Time: 20 minutes
Cooking Time: 45 minutes
Servings: 4

Ingredients

1 tablespoon fresh ginger
1 teaspoon oregano
1 teaspoon ground white pepper
1 teaspoon paprika
½ teaspoon soy sauce
1 teaspoon chili flakes
½ cup fresh basil
¼ lemon
3 tablespoon butter
2-pound halibut

Directions

1. Grate the fresh ginger and combine it with oregano, ground white pepper, and paprika, soy sauce and chili flakes in a large bowl. Stir to combine.

2. Slice the lemon.

3. Rub the halibut with the fresh ginger mixture and

put sliced lemon over the halibut.

4. Wrap the halibut in the fresh basil and put it in the plastic bag.

5. Preheat the water bath to 142°F/61°C and put the halibut there.

6. Cook fish for 45 minutes. When ready, remove fish from the bag and serve. Don't forget to discard the lemon and the basil.

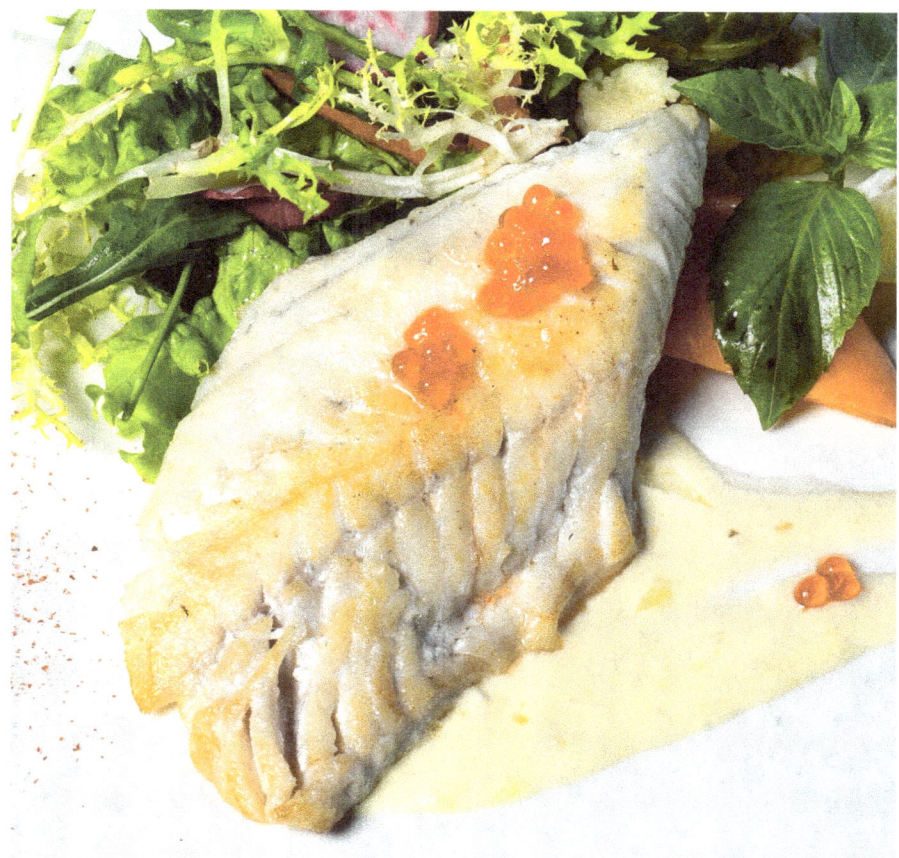

43. MEZCAL-LIME SHRIMP

Cal.: 389 | Fat: 32g | Protein: 16g

Preparation Time: 9 minutes
Cooking Time: 45 minutes
Servings: 4

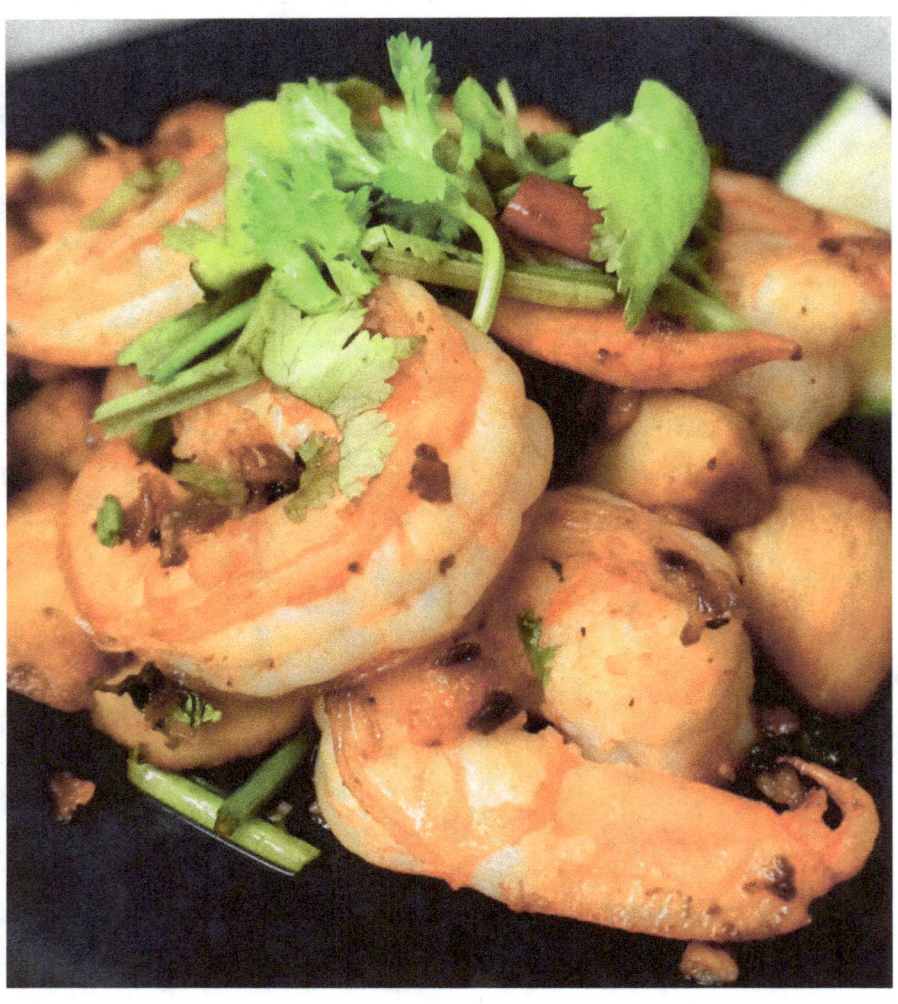

Ingredients

1 ½ pounds shell-on jumbo shrimp
1 oz. mezcal
Zest and juice of 1 lime
1 Tbsp. olive oil
1 tbsp. ancho chili powder
2 tsp. ground cumin
2 tsp. kosher salt
1 garlic clove, minced
Fresh cilantro, for serving

Directions

1. Preheat the water bath to 135°F/57°C.

2. Combine the shrimp, mezcal, olive oil, chili powder, lime zest, lime juice, cumin, salt and garlic in a large zipper-lock bag. Seal the bag using the water displacement method and place in the water bath.

3. Cook for 30 minutes, or up to 45 minutes.

4. Remove the bag from the water bath.

5. Pour the contents of the bag into a serving bowl and garnish with cilantro.

6. Serve.

44. POACHED TUNA WITH BASIL BUTTER

Cal.: 746 | Fat: 61.6g | Protein: 30.3g

Preparation Time: 15 minutes
Cooking Time: 27 minutes
Servings: 2

Ingredients

1 stick (½ cup) softened unsalted butter
1/3 cup fresh basil
2 garlic cloves
Zest of 1 lemon
Sea salt and freshly ground black pepper
2 7- ounce fresh tuna steaks, 1-inch thick
1-1 ½ cups extra virgin olive oil
Sea salt and freshly ground black pepper
2 tablespoons vegetable oil

Directions

1. Preheat the Sous Vide machine to 110°F/43°C. Finely mince the garlic and basil, and finely zest the lemon.

2. Mash together the butter with basil, garlic and lemon zest until well mixed. Add salt and pepper to taste.

3. Put each piece of tuna in a separate bag and pour in ½-3/4 cups of oil in each bag.

4. Place the bag in your preheated container and set your timer for 25 minutes.

5. While the salmon is cooking, place the butter on one side of a piece of plastic wrap. Roll the butter in the plastic wrap to create a log. Place the butter in the refrigerator.

6. When the tuna is almost cooked, heat the vegetable oil in a skillet over high heat. Remove the tuna from the bag and sear for 30 seconds per side.

7. Top with at least ½-inch-thick piece of basil butter to serve.

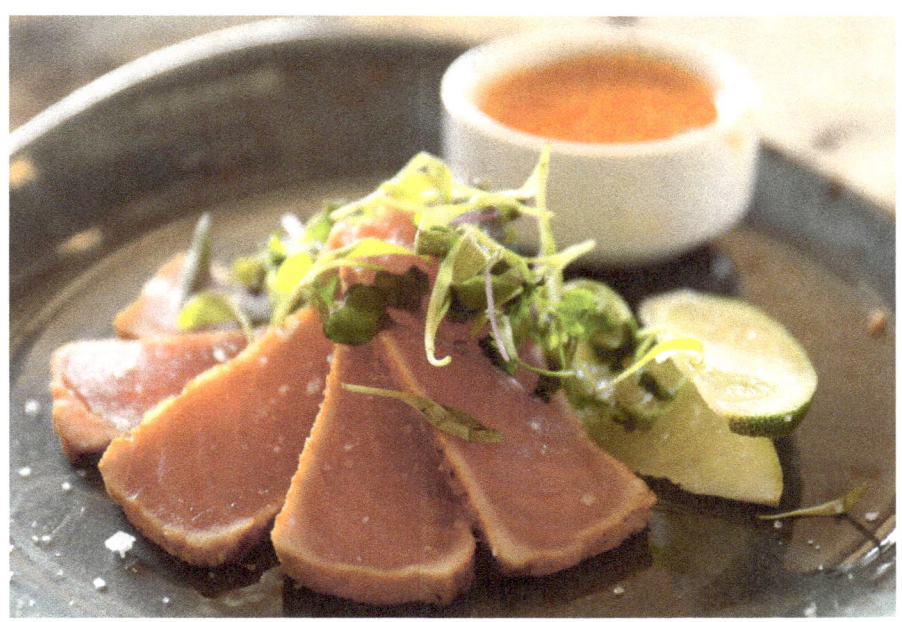

45. PECAN PIE

Cal.: 199 | Fat: 8g | Protein: 19g

Preparation Time: 9 minutes
Cooking Time: 2 hours 25 minutes
Servings: 8

Ingredients

1 cup maple syrup
2 cups of whole pecans
½ cup heavy cream
1 teaspoon Stevia sweetener
4 tbsp. unsalted butter
6 large egg yolks
½ tsp. salt
Freshly whipped cream

Directions

1. Preheat the Sous Vide machine to 195°F/91°C and preheat the oven to 350°F/176°C.

2. Prepare 8 ½-pint jars and grease the insides with butter or spray with cooking spray.

3. Place the pecan on a rimmed baking sheet and spread to make a single layer. Toast the pecans in the oven for 7–10 minutes. Once done, set aside

until cool enough to handle. Roughly chop the pecans and set aside.

4. In a medium saucepan, combine the molasses, heavy cream, stevia, and maple syrup. Set the saucepan over medium heat and stir the mixture until the stevia melts. Heat the mixture for 5 minutes while stirring continuously. Once done, remove the saucepan from the heat and let stand for 5 minutes.

5. Once the stevia mixture has cooled down, whisk the salt and butter into the saucepan until completely melted. Add in the egg yolks and whisk together until smooth. Add in the pecans and stir until evenly combined.

6. Divide the mixture evenly among the prepared jars, filling each jar halfway full. Clean the sides and tops of the jars using a damp towel.

7. Cover the jars with the lids as tight as you can with just using your fingertips to let a little bit of pressure escape and prevent the jars from exploding while cooking.

8. Place the jars in the water bath. Cook in the cooker for 2 hours.

9. Once done, remove the jars from the water bath and set on a wire rack. Remove the lids carefully and let cool to room temperature. To serve, top each pecan pie with whipped cream.

46. STRAWBERRY MOUSSE

Cal.: 265 | Fat: 4g | Protein: 17g

Preparation Time: 11 minutes
Cooking Time: 46 minutes
Servings: 4

Ingredients

1 pound strawberries, stemmed and halved
¼ teaspoon Stevia sweetener
3 tablespoons freshly squeezed lemon juice
½ teaspoon kosher salt
¼ teaspoon ground cinnamon
1 cup heavy cream
1 teaspoon vanilla extract
1 cup crème Fraîche

Directions

1. Prepare your water bath by dipping the immersion circulator and increasing the temperature to 180°F/82°C.

2. Add the strawberries, stevia, lemon juice, salt and cinnamon to a large-sized zip bag

3. Seal using the immersion method and cook for 45 minutes.

4. Remove the bag and transfer contents to a food processor.

5. Purée for a few seconds until you have a smooth mixture.

6. Take a large chilled mixing bowl and add heavy cream and vanilla; mix well until stiff peaks form.

7. Fold in strawberry purée and crème Fraiche.

8. Mix well and divide it among 8 serving bowls.

9. Serve chilled!

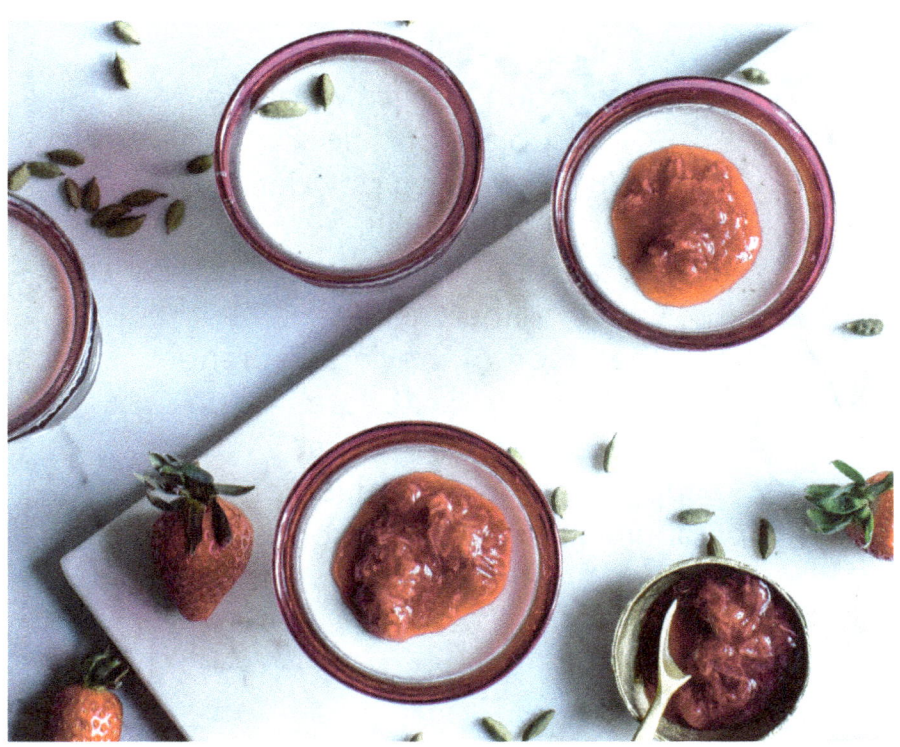

47. LEMON TART

Cal.: 273 | Fat: 4g | Protein: 12g

Preparation Time: 13 minutes
Cooking Time: 6 hours
Servings: 1

Ingredients

For the crust:
2 tbsp. cold water
1 egg yolk
1 cup keto flour
1 tsp. vanilla extract
1/3 teaspoon Stevia sweetener
¼ cup almond flour
1/8 tsp. baking powder
¼ tsp. salt
½ cup unsalted butter, cold and cubed
For the custard:
1 ½ teaspoon of Stevia Sweetener
8 egg yolks, beaten
2 tbsp. lemon zest
½ cup freshly squeezed lemon juice
1 ¾ cups of unsalted butter, at room temperature and cubed

Directions

1. To make the crust, set the oven to 375°F/190°C. Mix together the vanilla, cold water and egg yolk in a bowl. Add in the baking powder, salt, stevia, almond flour and all-purpose flour into the bowl and use an electric mixer to combine. While mixing, add in the butter cubes and continue to beat until smooth.

2. Form the dough into a bowl and cover using a plastic wrap. Chill in the refrigerator for 30 minutes. Once done, roll out the dough to make a thin sheet then place in a tart pan. Poke holes at the bottom using a fork. Bake the tart shell in the oven for 12 minutes or until the crust starts to brown. Once done, set aside to cool completely. To make the custard, preheat the Sous Vide machine to 149°F/65°C.

3. Place the egg yolks in a Ziploc bag and seal using the water immersion method. Place the bag into the water bath. Cook in the cooker for 35 minutes.

4. In a medium saucepan, combine the lemon juice and stevia and boil for 3 minutes or until the stevia is completely dissolved. Remove the saucepan from the heat and set aside to cool.

5. Once the eggs are done cooking, place the freezer bag into a bowl with ice and cold water. Then, pour the contents into a blender.

48. DARK CHOCOLATE MOUSSE

Cal.: 218 | Fat: 14g | Protein: 15g

Preparation Time: 11 minutes
Cooking Time: 31 hours
Servings: 4

Ingredients

2/3 cup dark chocolate, chopped
½ cup milk
½ cup double cream
½ tsp. gelatin powder
2 tbsp. cold water

Directions

1. Preheat the Sous Vide machine to 194°F/90°C.

2. Place the chopped dark chocolate in the vacuum bag.

3. Seal the bag, put it into the water bath and set the timer for 6 hours.

4. When the time is up, pour the chocolate into a bowl and stir with a spoon.

5. Pour the milk into a pan and warm it over medium heat.

6. Soak the gelatin powder in 2 tbsp. cold water and dissolve it in the warm milk.

7. Carefully stir the milk-gelatin mixture into the chocolate paste until even and refrigerate for 25 minutes.

8. Remove from the fridge, stir again and refrigerate for another 25 minutes.

9. Beat the cream to peaks and combine with white chocolate mixture.

10. Pour into single serve cups and refrigerate for 24 hours before serving.

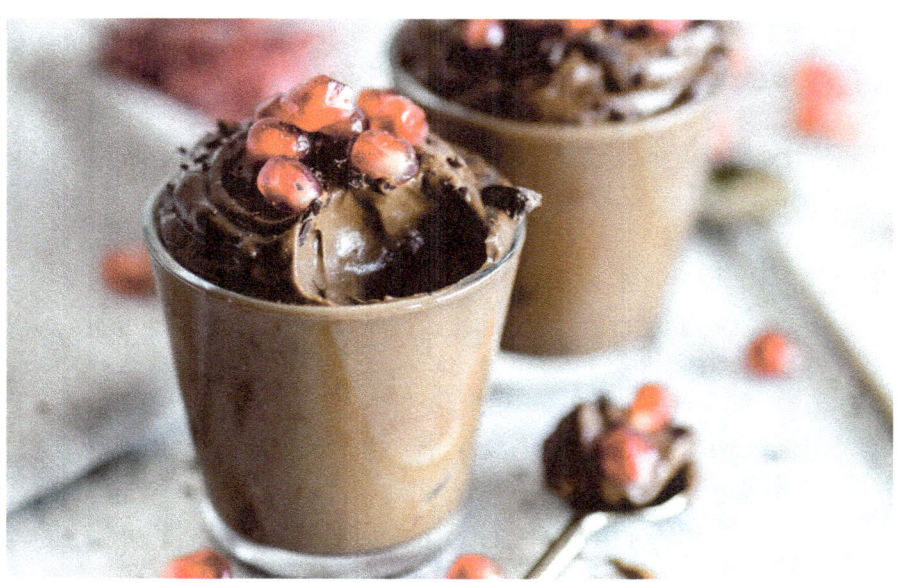

49. CRÈME BRÛLÉE

Cal.: 444 | Fat: 45.3g | Protein: 7g

Preparation Time: 2 hours 20 minutes
Cooking Time: 60 minutes
Servings: 6

Ingredients

11 egg yolks
Stevia sweentener
3 g salt
600 g heavy cream
6 (6-oz) mason jars

Directions

1. Preheat your Sous Vide Machine to 176°F/80°C.

2. Place the eggs, stevia and salt, in a bowl and whisk them together.

3. Carefully and slowly mix the cream into the egg mixture using a whisk. Otherwise, the eggs will curdle.

4. Strain the new mixture and allow it to rest for 20–30 minutes. The goal is to get rid of all the bubbles. Take off any removing bubbles.

5. Slowly pour an equal amount of the mixture from a low height into the mason jars. You want to make sure you don't create more bubbles.

6. Tighten the lids so they're finger tight. You don't want to tighten the lids as tight as possible, because the trapped air may crack the jars.

7. Place the jars in your preheated container and set your timer for 1 hour.

8. Once cooked, place the jars on a kitchen towel on the counter. Let the jars come down to room temperature.

9. Prepare an ice bath and place the cooled jars in the ice bath until cold.

10. Top the crème brulée with a layer of stevia using a sieve and use a kitchen torch to caramelize it. Allow it to harden for 5 minutes

11. Serve immediately.

50. MINI STRAWBERRY CHEESECAKE JARS

Cal.: 308 | Fat: 15g | Protein: 19g

Preparation Time: 8 minutes
Cooking Time: 90 minutes
Servings: 4

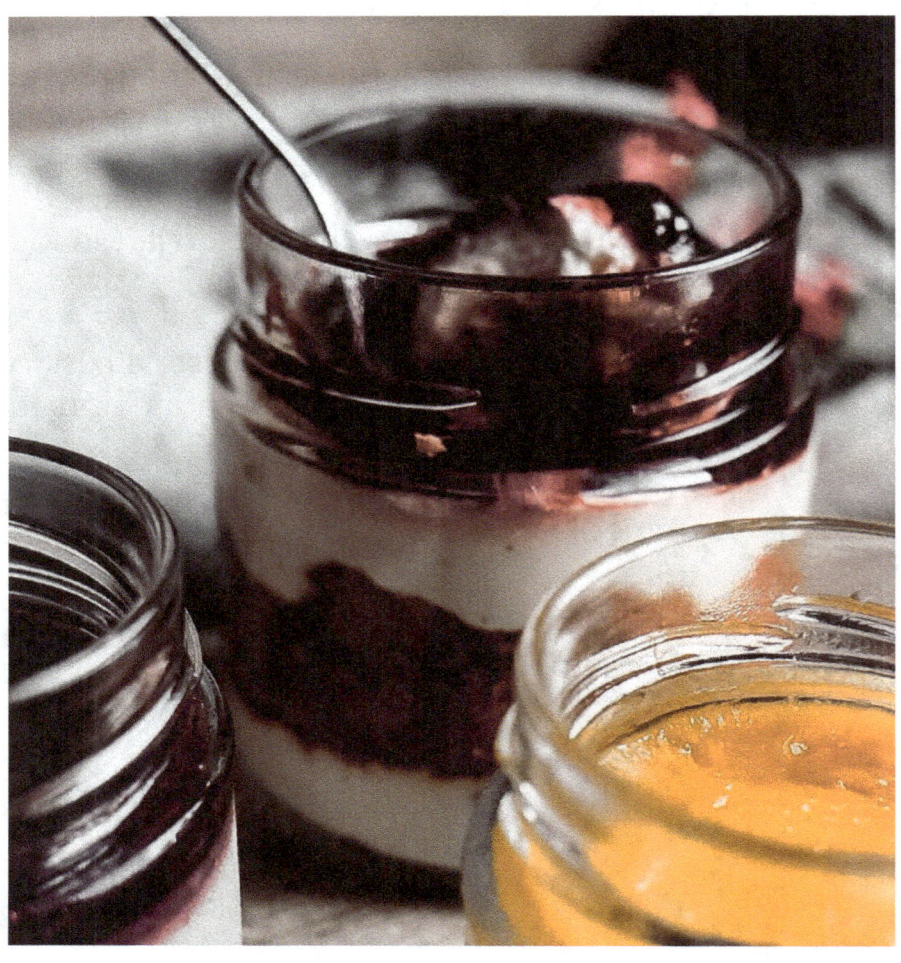

Ingredients

4 eggs
2 tbsp. milk
3 tbsp. strawberry jam
½ teaspoon Stevia sweetener
½ cup cream cheese
½ cup cottage cheese
1 tbsp. almond flour
1 tsp. lemon zest

Directions

1. Preheat the Sous Vide machine to 180°F/82°C. Beat together the cheeses and stevia until fluffy. Beat in the eggs, one by one.

2. Add the remaining ingredients and beat until well combined. Divide between 4 jars. Seal and place in the water. Cook for 75 minutes. Chill and serve.

TEMPERATURE CHARTS

🥩 MEAT	°F 🌡 TEMPERATURE	⏱ TIME
Beef Steak, rare	129 °F	1 hour 30 min.
Beef Steak, medium-rare	136 °F	1 hour 30min.
Beef Steak, well done	158 °F	1 hour 30min.
Beef Roast, rare	133 °F	7 hours
Beef Roast, medium-rare	140 °F	6 hours
Beef Roast, well done	158 °F	5 hours
Beef Tough Cuts, rare	136 °F	24 hours
Beef Tough Cuts, medium-rare	149 °F	16 hours
Beef Tough Cuts, well done	185 °F	8 hours
Lamb Tenderloin, Rib eye, T-bone, Cutlets	134 °F	4 hours
Lamb Roast, Leg	134 °F	10 hours
Lamb Flank Steak, Brisket	134 °F	12 hours
Pork Chop, rare	136 °F	1 hour
Pork Chop, medium-rare	144 °F	1 hour
Pork Chop, well done	158 °F	1 hour
Pork Roast, rare	136 °F	3 hours

🥩 MEAT	🌡 TEMPERATURE	⏱ TIME
Pork Roast, medium-rare	144 °F	3 hours
Pork Roast, well done	158 °F	3 hours
Pork Tough Cuts, rare	144 °F	16 hours
Pork Tough Cuts, medium-rare	154 °F	12 hours
Pork Tough Cuts, well done	154 °F	8 hours
Pork Tenderloin	134 °F	1 hour 30min
Pork Baby Back Ribs	165 °F	6 hours
Pork Cutlets	134 °F	5 hours
Pork Spare Ribs	160 °F	12 hours
Pork Belly (quick)	185 °F	5 hours
Pork Belly (slow)	167 °F	24 hours

🐟 FISH AND SEAFOOD	🌡 TEMPERATURE	⏱ TIME
Fish, tender	104 °F	40 min.
Fish, tender and flaky	122 °F	40 min.
Fish, well done	140 °F	40 min.
Salmon, Tuna, Trout, Mackerel, Halibut, Snapper, Sole	126 °F	30 min.
Lobster	140 °F	50 min.
Scallops	140 °F	50 min.
Shrimp	140 °F	35 min.

🍗 POULTRY	°F 🌡 TEMPERATURE	⏱ TIME
Chicken White Meat, super-supple	140 °F	2 hours
Chicken White Meat, tender and juicy	149 °F	1 hour
Chicken White Meat, well done	167 °F	1 hour
Chicken Breast, bone-in	146 °F	2 hours 30 min.
Chicken Breast, boneless	146 °F	1 hour
Turkey Breast, bone-in	146 °F	4 hours
Turkey Breast, boneless	146 °F	2 hours 30 min.
Duck Breast	134 °F	1 hour 30 min.
Chicken Dark Meat, tender	149 °F	1 hour 30 min.
Chicken Dark Meat, falling off the bone	167 °F	1 hour 30 min.
Chicken Leg or Thigh, bone-in	165 °F	4 hours
Chicken Thigh, boneless	165 °F	1 hour
Turkey Leg or Thigh	165 °F	2 hours
Duck Leg	165 °F	8 hours
Split Game Hen	150 °F	6 hours

🥕 VEGETABLES	°F TEMPERATURE	⏱ TIME
Vegetables, root (carrots, potato, parsnips, beets, celery root, turnips)	183 °F	3 hours
Vegetables, tender (asparagus, broccoli, cauliflower, fennel, onions, pumpkin, eggplant, green beans, corn)	183 °F	1 hour
Vegetables, greens (kale, spinach, collard greens, Swiss chard)	183 °F	3 min.

🍎 FRUITS	°F TEMPERATURE	⏱ TIME
Fruit, firm (apple, pear)	183 °F	45 min.
Fruit, for purée	185 °F	30 min.
Fruit, berries for topping desserts (blueberries, blackberries, raspberries, strawberries, cranberries)	154 °F	30 min.

WHAT TEMPERATURE SHOULD BE USED?

The rule of thumb is that the thicker the piece, the longer it should cook. Higher temperatures shorten the cooking time. Lower temperatures may take longer.

	TEMPERATURE	MIN COOKING TIME	MAX COOKING TIME
EGGS			
Soft Yolk	140°F (60°C)	1 hour	1 hour
Creamy Yolk	145°F (63°C)	¾ hour	1 hour
GREEN VEGETABLES			
Rare	183°F (84°C)	¼ hour	¾ hour
ROOTS			
Rare	183°F (84°C)	1 hour	3 hours
FRUITS			
Warm	154°F (68°C)	1¾ hour	2½ hour
Soft Fruits	185°F (85°C)	½ hour	1½ hour

	TEMPERATURE	MIN COOKING TIME	MAX COOKING TIME
CHICKEN			
Rare	140°F (60°C)	1 hour	3 hours
Medium	150°F (65°C)	1 hour	3 hours
Well Done	167°F (75°C)	1 hour	3 hours
BEEF STEAK			
Rare	130°F (54°C)	1½ hours	3 hours
Medium	140°F (60°C)	1½ hours	3 hours
Well Done	145°F (63°C)	1½ hours	3 hours
ROAST BEEF			
Rare	133°F (54°C)	7 hours	16 hours
Medium	140°F (60°C)	6 hours	14 hours
Well Done	158°F (70°C)	5 hours	11 hours
PORK CHOP BONE-IN			
Rare	136°F (58°C)	1 hour	4 hours
Medium	144°F (62°C)	1 hour	4 hours
Well Done	158°F (70°C)	1 hour	4 hours
PORK LOIN			
Rare	136°F (58°C)	3 hours	5½ hours
Medium	144°F (62°C)	3 hours	5 hours
Well Done	158°F (70°C)	3 hours	3½ hours
FISH			
Tender	104°F (40°C)	½ hour	½ hour
Medium	124°F (51°C)	½ hour	1 hour
Well Done	131°F (55°C)	½ hour	1½ hours

COOKING CONVERSION

TEMPERATURE CONVERSIONS	
CELSIUS	**FAHRENHEIT**
54.5°C	130°F
60.0°C	140°F
65.5°C	150°F
71.1°C	160°F
76.6°C	170°F
82.2°C	180°F
87.8°C	190°F
93.3°C	200°F
100°C	212°F

WEIGHT COVERSION	
½ oz.	15g
1 oz.	30g
2 oz.	60g
3 oz.	85g
4 oz.	110g
5 oz.	140g
6 oz.	170g
7 oz.	200g
8 oz.	225g
9 oz.	255g
10 oz.	280g
11 oz.	310g
12 oz.	340g
13 oz.	370g
14 oz.	400g
15 oz.	425g
1 lb.	450g

LIQUID VOLUME CONVERSION		
CUPS / TABLESPOONS	FL. OUNCES	MILLILITERS
1 cup	8 fl. Oz.	240 ml
¾ cup	6 fl. Oz.	180 ml
2/3 cup	5 fl. Oz.	150 ml
½ cup	4 fl. Oz.	120 ml
1/3 cup	2 ½ fl. Oz.	75 ml
¼ cup	2 fl. Oz.	60 ml
1/8 cup	1 fl. Oz.	30 ml
1 tablespoon	½ fl. Oz.	15 ml

TEASPOON (tsp.) / TABLESPOON (Tbsp.)	MILLILITERS
1 tsp.	5ml
2 tsp.	10ml
1 Tbsp.	15ml
2 Tbsp.	30ml
3 Tbsp.	45ml
4 Tbsp.	60ml
5 Tbsp.	75ml
6 Tbsp.	90ml
7 Tbsp.	105ml

LIQUID VOLUME MEASUREMENTS				
TABLE-SPOONS	TEASPOONS	FLUID OUNCES	CUPS
16	48	8 fl. Oz.	1
12	36	6 fl. Oz.	¾
8	24	4 fl. Oz.	½
5 ½	16	2 2/3 fl. Oz.	1/3
4	12	2 fl. Oz.	¼
1	3	0.5 fl. Oz.	1/16

RECIPE INDEX

Asparagus with Hollandaise 39
Baked Yam Chips 12
Cauliflower 14
Cauliflower Soup 46
Chicken Skewers 24
Chili and Garlic Sauce 78
Chipotle Apple Pork Loin 58
Cider Dipped Fennel 42
Cinnamon and Egg Mix 43
Cream of Celery Soup 18
Crème Brûlée 102
Dark Chocolate Mousse 100
Egg 38
Eggs with Roasted Peppers 36
Favorite Thai Dinner 50
Flank Steak, Apricot, and Brie Bites 16
Flax Seeds Mix 40
French Duck Confit 60
Fresh Vegetables Confit 28
Garlic Dipping Sauce with Asparagus 82
Herbed Pork Chops 20
Indian Style Pork 68
Lamb Chops with Basil Chimichurri 56
Lemongrass and Garlic Pork Belly Roll 26

Lemon Tart	98
Mezcal-Lime Shrimp	90
Mid-Week Chicken	52
Mini Strawberry Cheesecake Jars	104
Miso Soy Glazed Pork Chops	66
Okra and Spiced Yogurt	30
Parmesan and Scallion Omelet	32
Parmesan Garlic Asparagus	76
Pecan Pie	94
Perfect Egg Tostada	34
Perfectly Cooked Mushrooms	72
Poached Tuna with Basil Butter	92
Pork Chops with Mushrooms	48
Pork Tenderloin	54
Sausage Tomato	62
Savory Halibut	88
Scallops with Lemon Herb Salsa Verde	84
Simple Mushroom Soup	44
Soft-Poached Eggs	35
Spice Rubbed Short Ribs	64
Strawberry Mousse	96
Swordfish with Balsamic Brown Butter Sauce	86
Tender Leeks with Herbed Butter	74
Tomatoes Stuffed with Tuna	22
Turmeric Pickled Cauliflower	80
Warm Beef Soup with Ginger	70

www.ingramcontent.com/pod-product-compliance
Lightning Source LLC
Chambersburg PA
CBHW070925080526
44589CB00013B/1427